# 30-Day Body Purifcation

## HOW TO CLEANSE YOUR INNER BODY & EXPERIENCE THE JOYS OF TOXIN-FREE HEALTH

## Lewis

WITH

PREN
Paramus

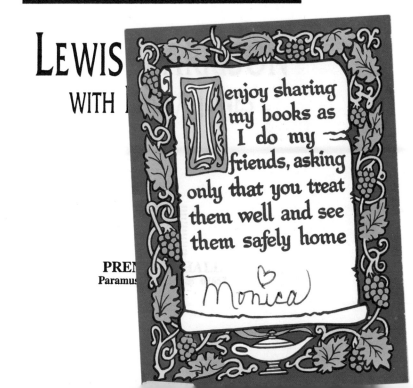

I enjoy sharing my books as I do my friends, asking only that you treat them well and see them safely home

Monica

*Printed in the United States of America*

*10  9  8  7  6  5  4  3  2  1        10  9  8  7  6  5  4*

ISBN 0-13-917253-X    ISBN 0-13-917303-X (PBK)

This book is reference work based on research by the author. The opinions expressed herein are not necessarily those of or endorsed by the publisher. The directions stated in this book are in no way to be considered as a substitute for consultation with a duly licensed doctor.

---

**ATTENTION: CORPORATIONS AND SCHOOLS**

Parker Publishing Company books are available at quantity discounts with bulk purchase for educational, business, or sales promotional use. For information, please write to: Prentice Hall Career & Personal Development Special Sales, 240 Frisch Court, Paramus, NJ 076532. Please supply: title of book, ISBN number, quantity, how the book will be used, date needed.

---

**PARKER PUBLISHING COMPANY**
West Nyack, NY 10994

A Simon & Schuster Company

On the World Wide Web at http://www.phdirect.com

Prentice-Hall International (UK) Limited, *London*
Prentice-Hall of Australia Pty. Limited, *Sydney*
Prentice-Hall Canada Inc., *Toronto*
Prentice-Hall Hispanoamericana, S.A., *Mexico*
Prentice-Hall of India Private Limited, *New Delhi*
Prentice-Hall of Japan, Inc., *Tokyo*
Simon & Schuster Asia Pte. Ltd., *Singapore*
Editora Prentice-Hall do Brasil, Ltda., *Rio de Janeiro*

# DEDICATION

To Martin Kalmanson, Vincent Collura and Maharaj Charan Singh. My three closest friends and teachers who passed away during the writing of this book. They lived full and joyous lives. I deeply miss their laughter.

# ACKNOWLEDGMENT

Writing a book is a team project. Consequently there are many people to thank for making this book a reality. First I would like to thank Jeff Wolf, Michael Campbell, Mark Becker, Martin Ravitsky, Dr. James Lynch, Linda Collura, Janice Latham, and Sid Jainchill for their emotional and financial support. It gave me the freedom to gather the necessary research material. I would like to express my appreciation to my associates, staff, students, research interns, and word processors including Tanya Mammon, Gloria Santos, Russell Feingold, Shelley Pederson, Adam Whyte and Ann Held, for going beyond "the call of duty" to help make this book a reality. I also want to thank my editor at Prentice-Hall, Doug Corcoran for keeping the book alive and to my agent Rita Rosenkranz for her guidance and support. I would also like to thank my mother Dorothy Harrison who taught me to finish what you start.

I know for certain that there would not be a book without my co-author Laura Jones. Laura organized the program into a superbly written, easy-to-follow format. In addition she worked overtime on a tight deadline and did it with a smile and enthusiastic spirit.

# TABLE OF CONTENTS

## 4. WEEK #2: LIGHTEN UP WITH GENTLE JUICE CLEANSING 53

## 5. WEEK #3: FASTING FOR OPTIMAL HEALTH   77

## 6. WEEK #4: REBUILDING YOUR NEW HEALTHY BODY   91

## 7. MAINTAINING YOUR HEALTHY BODY   115

# WHAT THIS BOOK CAN DO FOR YOU

As a teacher, writer, and consultant for many years on health, I have repeatedly been asked by readers, students, clients, physicians, and practitioners of various healing arts to compile a set of guidelines that would assist in the promotion of detoxification, healing, and rejuvenation of the mind and body. While gathering research for my previous publications, I compiled this and used it in my classes. Over the years, many of my colleagues suggested that I turn this compilation of information into a book. They were excited about such a project because it would fill a modern health need by clarifying the confusion that so many people have about juice diets, weight-loss programs, appetite reduction, fasting, and so on by offering specific purification techniques for tackling various health problems and ridding the body of chemical toxins.

This book is a unique guide for anyone who not only wants relief from ill health, but also wants to regain a sense of well-being. By following my suggestions you will experience greater vigor, and also maintain a youthful appearance and generally get more out of living.

In organizing this book, I had three objectives: to improve your health on a daily basis, to save you from a potentially crippling or fatal disease resulting from internal toxification, and to prolong your life.

The information offered here is based on 22 years of extensive research and clinical experience as a consultant to holistic doctors and wellness specialists.

In my opinion, these are the most effective approaches yet known to prevent and treat internal toxicity, which, along with genetic factors is the greatest cause of sickness and death.

At this very moment, research scientists and physicians all over the world are searching for the "magic pills" that will cure our physical and emotional ills. Until the day that this knowledge arrives, I believe we should use the most perfect tools that we now have, namely, the body purification tools presented and described in this book. The mounting evidence that eating the proper foods combined, with juicing, fasting, supplementation, and exercise can save the health and lives of millions is now too powerful to allow us to wait for the perfect cure or a magic pill.

If you read this book carefully, and follow the simple, easy-to-apply directions given, it is my belief that you will be able to.

## 1. IMMEDIATELY IMPROVE YOUR HEALTH

Whether it's maintaining trouble-free digestion, reducing arthritis pain, eliminating menstrual cramps, increasing mental and physical stamina, having more youthful skin, reducing allergic reactions, increasing your ability to relax and to sleep restfully or simply controlling your weight, following this program will bring immediate results. Many researchers agree that the combination of a purifying diet, increased fiber, a reduced intake of sugar and salt, exercise, and stress management can produce dramatic improvements in those who seem to have the greatest health problems.

## 2. KNOW WHAT FOODS TO EAT AND WHEN

*The 30-Day Body Purification Program* will prolong your life by cleansing your blood stream and internal organs. In the following pages you will be instructed step by step on what to eat to maintain an effective cleansing program. The program provides complete and detailed menus for breakfast, lunch, and dinner for a full 30 days. It also provides recipes and food shopping guidance week by week. Special sections are included on beans, grains, and herbs, including special cleansing herbal tea recipes.

## 3. GROW YOUNGER THROUGH THE MAGIC OF FOOD SUPPLEMENTATION

Medical science has discovered many important nutritional supplements that not only improve your general health but can even remove toxic substances from your body. Many of these toxic substances can cause cancer and heart disease.

The supplements described in the following pages can help you overcome fatigue, stress, loss of energy, and sluggish circulation.

Modern science has amply demonstrated that millions of Americans eat throughout the day and yet they are still poorly nourished. They suffer from all the symptoms of nutritional deficiency disorders. The 30-Day Body Purification Program integrates these important supplements into the 30 day menu.

## 4. PUT HEALTH AND JOY IN EVERY DAY OF YOUR LIFE THROUGH THE BODY/MIND APPROACH

Modern science now knows that what affects the body also affects the mind and vice versa. I believe that, in addition to a purifying nutrition program, proper exercise, rest, relaxation visualization exercises, and stress management will enable you to gain added years to your life. These are years of health that otherwise could have the potential to be filled with unhappiness and ill health.

Each step of the program is listed plainly to assist you in organizing your complete purifying and health building program. The program includes tasty, nutritional recipes of ordinary fruits, vegetables, nuts, seeds, grains, herbs, spices, and enzyme-rich cultured dairy products like yogurt and buttermilk. Specific suggestions and guidelines are offered for using juice therapy and simple, inexpensive nutritional supplements, such as vitamins, minerals, amino acids, and herbs. These will help you to reduce toxin buildup in your body. Other simple guidelines for hydrotherapy and self-massage techniques are offered for increasing and revitalizing sluggish circulation. The unique benefit of this book is that these suggestions are so easy, require only a few moments, and are totally cost free, as no special products or tools are needed. Each technique you apply will help revitalize your body and increase your feeling of aliveness.

# WHAT IS BODY PURIFICATION?

The amazing discovery of body purification came about when researchers discovered that sick people could become healthy again when they learned to remove toxins from their bodies. While medical treatment usually battles disease after it occurs, body purification aims to remove the cause of disease before we become ill.

Under normal conditions your immune system, utilizing each organ of elimination, will maintain a healthy and balanced internal environment. Under the abnormal conditions of stress created by an unhealthy lifestyle and the intake of toxic substances, these organs become loaded with systemic poisons. This toxic overloading radically alters the internal ecosystem of your body, encouraging the growth of bacteria, parasites, and other microorganisms that can lead to inflammatory and other disease processes.

When we look at the environmental causes of disease, we can see that the human body is much like a garden. Just as a garden with poor top soil cannot produce healthy plants, so illness and disease are growths that feed on poisoned soil. To thrive, a garden needs nutrients, water, and a growing environment of healthy rich topsoil Your body needs a healthy environment as well.

The basic goal of body purification is to cleanse the body's internal ecosystem of toxic metabolic wastes and other clogging substances that have resulted from eating highly processed, denatured food, breathing poor air, drinking tainted water, and living under artificial light and emotional stress. Cleansing with herbs and pure nutrients are the keys to restoring a healthy, nourishing environment in and around the body.

The concept of body purification has been a major healing technique for thousands of years in many cultures. Herbal purification fasting has been used by Native Americans for hundreds of years, and many communities continue to practice ceremonies celebrating its use for physical, mental, and spiritual purification.

*The 30-Day Body Purification Program* is a unique guide for anyone who wants relief from ill health, to regain a sense of well being, experience, greater vigor, and generally to get more out of living .

Creating trouble-free digestion, reducing arthritis pain, eliminating menstrual cramps, increasing mental stamina, having more youthful skin, reducing many allergic reactions, increasing the ability to relax and to sleep well, eliminating chemical toxins from your body, and reducing your appetite are just a few of the benefits possible through following this program.

The program is presented step by step. Some of the steps require ordinary fruits and vegetables. Others call for juices or water. Specific suggestions and guidelines are offered for using inexpensive nutritional supplements such as vitamins, minerals, amino acids, and herbs to reduce toxin buildup in your body. Other simple guidelines for hydrotherapy, stretching, yoga postures, and self-massage techniques are offered for increasing and revitalizing sluggish circulation. These purifying and health-building techniques are easy to use, requiring only a few moments each day, and many are free, requiring no special products or tools. Let the 30-day program work for you and learn what being truly healthy can mean!

# CONQUER TOXIC OVERLOAD WITH BODY PURIFICATION

## HOW TOXIC OVERLOAD MAKES YOU SICK

Everything that exists, whether natural or artificial, is composed of chemicals — food, clothing, even you and I. Consider, for example, a fresh orange. Ascorbic acid, inositol, biotin, tartaric acid, choline, nucleotides, and peroxidase are just a few of the chemicals that make up this fruit! These complex words may be unfamiliar to you, but they are routine names used by scientists to describe the chemical substances found everywhere in nature. Unfortunately, many food manufacturers feel that the chemicals chosen by Mother Nature are inadequate and that it is necessary to add synthetic chemical compounds, otherwise known as "additives" to foods during processing. When you choose highly processed foods, the flavor, aroma, and texture you experience are created through the use of these synthetic, non-nutritional additives. Highly processed denatured foods may look good, smell good, and taste good, but they really are a chemical feast. The false appearance, flavor, and texture of freshness have been created by processing body-polluting additives into foods that are no longer actually fresh.

Because your body does not require and cannot make use of these additives, it must neutralize and eliminate them from its system. This task of detoxification requires energy that you are supposed to be getting from the food you eat. If your diet is high in processed foods, your body is not getting the nutritional energy it needs. In this diminished state, body polluting additives do not get eliminated and instead build up to toxic levels. Eventually, this toxic overload will create disease somewhere in your body. It is actually possible to eat yourself sick!

## FOOD POLLUTION: GET THE JUNK OUT OF YOUR FOOD TODAY!

There are many levels to food processing, and the fact that a food has been minced, heated, canned, frozen, or altered in other ways does not necessarily make it a poor food choice. It is when synthetic additives come into play that the problem begins.

Unnecessary artificial additives may take the form of:

> Emulsifiers
> Preservatives
> Flavor enhancers (e.g., M.S.G. — monosodium glutamate)
> Artificial flavors
> Artificial colors

Manufacturers add these chemicals instead of using natural ingredients because they are cheaper. But artificial additives are not really necessary. You can create delicious, appealing healthy dishes in your kitchen by using fresh organically grown ingredients.

### EMULSIFIERS—BEWARE OF THREE UNDESIRABLES

By nature, some liquids, for example, oil and water, will not mix. The addition of emulsifiers permits liquids to blend and remain stable or "emulsify."

Great-grandmother found that her baked goods were finer in texture and the grain had greater volume when she added eggs to her cake batter. Eggs allowed an even blending of fat with liquids and air that went into making the batter. Today, emulsifiers are most frequently used to improve the texture of commercially processed baked goods, but they also keep the oils blended in foods such as ice cream, frozen desserts, pourable salad dressings, and chocolate. For example, the smooth uniform texture of ice cream and similar frozen desserts depends, in part, on emulsifiers that permit the complete blending of ingredients.

Undesirable emulsifiers to watch out for include: calcium salts, acetate, and diacetate.

The best emulsifier is lecithin, which is made from soybeans.

## PRESERVATIVES—CREATE YOUR OWN

In the past, without the aid of refrigeration, our ancestors were forced to hunt and gather food early in the morning for their daily meals. To preserve food for future meals, sugar was added to fruit, meat was coated with salt, and pickles were preserved in a vinegar solution.

Today, salt and sugar are still used to control the growth of organisms that cause spoilage. In addition, there are now synthetically produced preservatives that inhibit or prevent the growth of microorganisms in food such as bread, shortening, and fruit juices. In spite of what food manufacturers might imply, natural forms of preservation in food processing are still applicable. Health food stores are filled with processed foods that have been vacuum packed, canned, or frozen without artificial preservatives.

One of the first types of food spoilage is discoloration. When some foods such as apples or peaches are cut, the exposed surface turns brown. In the past, cooks often dipped sliced fruit in lemon, orange, lime or pineapple juice to prevent discoloration. With discoloration there is often a change in flavor. This is caused by the oxygen in the air reacting with the juices of the cut fruit.

When spoilage takes place in a fat or oil, it will appear as a distasteful odor or flavor. These changes are the result of oxidation. Since lard and other edible fats were very difficult to store for an extended period, they were rendered and filtered to remove impurities. Then they were stored in the coolest spot available to prevent them from rapidly turning rancid.

Today, antioxidants are used in canning and freezing to preserve the color of the food. Fats are still filtered and clarified, but we also have antioxidants that prevent or delay oxidative changes in processed foods containing fats and oils, such as baking mixes, margarine, mayonnaise, salad dressing, and shortening.

In your healthy kitchen, you will want to dip sliced fruit in lemon, orange, lime or pineapple juice to maintain the fruit's appealing color. Purchase oils in dark glass bottles and keep them in your refrigerator. Open a vitamin E gel capsule and squeeze the oil into any food containing vegetable oils (dressings, batters, etcetera), properly seal and refrigerate all perishables, and scan all product labels carefully for artificial preservatives such as calcium proprionate and sodium proprionate.

## FLAVORINGS—NATURE KNOWS BEST

Flavor is an important factor in determining whether or not a food is acceptable. No matter how nutritious or attractive a food may be, if the flavor is unappealing, it will probably not be eaten! For this reason, flavoring agents are the largest and most diverse group of food additives. Synthetic flavoring agents are the flavor of choice if you are going to create an artificial food that will never mold, never need to be refrigerated, has had all the enzymes and most of the nutrients destroyed in processing, and has had synthetic vitamins added back in! The more processed and denatured a food is, the more it requires uniform, cheap flavorings.

Watch out for synthetic flavorings and flavor enhancers (such as M.S.G.). These chemicals have no nutritional value and serve only to mask the poor flavor quality of an overprocessed food. Many people have strong allergic reactions to M.S.G., giving all of us an additional reason to avoid this unnecessary additive.

Our forebears found that flavorings and spices made their foods more palatable, added variety to routine foods, and made mealtime a pleasure rather than a necessity. As you become familiar with the 30-Day Body Purification Program recipes, you will discover how herbs and spices such as cinnamon, chili, and vanilla can make your healthy food a joy to prepare and serve.

## COLOR ENHANCERS—AVOID THE FAKES

For appetite appeal, it is important that foods have characteristic and attractive colors. In processing or cooking foods, changes occur that require the addition of a coloring agent to recapture the characteristic color.

Today, people have become accustomed to foods made almost entirely of additives, for example, a fruit pudding that contains no fruit. The characteristic colors we associate with different flavors of gelatin desserts, puddings, soft drinks, frozen desserts, and prepared mixes are provided almost entirely by synthetic coloring agents. More than 90 percent are synthetically produced, while the others are derived from plants. Natural foods are colored in much the same way as they were in the past, when our forefathers used beet juice, crushed parsley, saffron, paprika, and berries to give their foods an appealing color.

## REMOVE ADDITIVES TO REDUCE HYPERACTIVITY IN CHILDREN

Studies have shown that chemical additives, especially artificial flavors and colors, in processed convenience-type foods are a cause of learning and behavior problems in children. Much of the clinical research on this was done by a prominent allergist, the late Dr. Ben Feingold, of the Kaiser-Permanente Medical Group, in San Francisco. Dr. Feingold discovered that much hyperactivity could be traced to what are known as salicylates, which, in addition to being a component of various drugs, also occur naturally in foods and are used in many additives, especially as artificial colorings and artificial flavorings. Salicylates are found in antioxidants, leaveners, thickeners, and an endless list of additives. Many hyperkinetic children are extremely sensitive to these chemicals and will react to them. It is important for the parents of these children to teach them about the offending agents so that they can avoid them.

The 30-Day Purification Program is extremely helpful to these hyperactive children. When salicylates are removed from the diet of many hyperactive children, says Dr. Feingold, they're well on their way to "normal" behavior and often show "increased scholastic ability within a month's time. Many of these children have high I.Q.s, but hyperkinesis tends to disrupt their attention span and learning process."

Even natural sources of salicylates should be removed from the diet. These foods include wine, wine vinegar, grapes, apricots, tomatoes, plums, berries, and tea. A complete list of salicylate rich foods can be found in Dr. Feingold's book, *An Introduction to Clinical Allergy* (Charles C. Thomas, 1973).

*The 30-Day Purification Program will*

1. Clean out the chemical additives that have built up in your system
2. Teach you new and improved ways of eating
3. Help you avoid creating future health problems
4. Increase your energy levels and sense of well being.

And now let's consider your home and office environment and see what positive changes we can make to limit your exposure to health-robbing materials and influences.

## CLEARING THE AIR: ELIMINATE POLLUTION AT YOUR OFFICE AND IN YOUR HOME

One of the contributing factors to poor health that we seldom think about is indoor pollution. According to a report in the medical magazine, *Geriatrics* (Vol. 46, no. 1, January 1991), "the workplace environment is dominated by man-made hazards: asbestos, organic solvents and oils, plastics, repetitive trauma, noise pollution, vibration, welding fumes, fibrous glass, and lead. These hazards are associated with various diseases and disabilities, such as hearing loss, asthma, carpal tunnel syndrome, sleep disturbances associated with shift work, and occupational stress."

Your home environment is also probably not as safe as you think it is. The danger? Chemical pollution! Just look at the labels on the products you keep under your kitchen or bathroom sink. Directions for common household products often warn against inhalation or direct contact with skin.

*Eleven Hazardous Indoor Chemical Pollutants:*

1. Odors and fumes from gas appliances (especially from a gas stove)
2. The combustion products of gas, oil, or coal
3. Insecticides
4. Refrigerants
5. Certain plastics
6. Hair sprays
7. Paints, primers and thinners (may emit toxic fumes and odors from fungicides for years)

8. Disinfectants

9. Shellac (can cause reactions if you are chemically allergic to oils- and solvent-based finishes and/or synthetics)

10. Spackles and other adhesive products (can contain fumes of softeners, solvents, and other additives)

11. Shoe polish and household cleaners (Many people are now aware that conventional shoe polish can contain up to seven highly toxic ingredients, one being methylene chloride. The inhalation of these vapors can cause carbon monoxide accumulation in the blood stream.)

These chemical agents can be a cause of mental disturbances dependent upon individual susceptibility to buildup from multiple exposures. Symptomatic reactions range from mental confusion and physical and/or mental fatigue to depression and advance psychotic states.

## WHAT YOU CAN DO NOW ABOUT INDOOR POLLUTION AT HOME

If you have a healthy life-style and become ill, see a holistically oriented physician or health consultant. If no specific diagnosis can be made, look into the possibility that you may be reacting to some environmental pollutants.

While investigating the cause of your health problem, pay attention to any unusual or new health problems that you may be experiencing. And be sure to keep a log of dates and particulars, and investigate the environment of your home or place of work.

### *Healthy Alternative Products*

*Oil Finishes/Preservatives:* Many exterior wood preservatives contain highly toxic creosote or arsenics. There are water-resistant exterior preservative products available that are non-polluting and effective. These products contain elastic qualities that allow the wood to breathe while preventing peel-offs or bubbles.

*Shellac:* An acceptable shellac should contain quick evaporation alcohol as a solvent. This is especially important if you are environmentally sensitive to oil- and solvent-based finishes and/or synthetics.

*Spackles/Adhesives:* Fumes of softeners, solvents, and other additives in conventional adhesives make these products unacceptable if you are chemically sensitive or want to avoid inhalable chemicals.

*Paints/Primers/Thinners:* Many products emit toxic fumes and odors from fungicides for years. Look for products that contain only the pure fragrances of natural plant extracts and essential oils. Once the paint is completely dry, no fumes should be emitted into the atmosphere.

*Cleaner/Polish:* The inhalation of the vapors in these products can cause carbon monoxide accumulation in the bloodstream. Look for products made with herbal extract, natural tree resins, and pure spirits (alcohols derived form beets or potatoes), and be sure to provide plenty of ventilation of fresh air whenever you clean.

NOTE: *When using products that claim to be safe for chemically sensitive people or extremely allergic people, it is a good idea to do a test prior to covering large areas and to consult your clinical ecologist. Ingredients should be listed on the product labels. When using any products that produce fumes or a strong odor, be sure that rooms are well ventilated during application. It is advisable (especially when covering large areas) to have additional protection with carbon-filter masks as well as gloves.*

For a list of non-allergic, non-polluting products contact:
LIVOS PRODUCTS
2641 Cerillos Road
Santa Fe, NM 87501
(505) 988-9111

## CLEARING THE OFFICE AIR

In addition to eliminating toxic chemicals from the home and office, there are many things that you can do to improve your environment. Of greatest importance is the circulation of clean air. In many companies there is no circulation of clean air because they have closed off the air vents. This may be done in an overzealous effort to conserve energy. This stale air is commonly called "blue haze." When air is stale, workers get drowsy and became less productive. (In a Virginia bank vents that had been sealed for two years were opened, and the stale air problem disappeared as if by magic!)

Much attention has been placed in recent years on the problem that cigarette smoke poses to clean air in the work place. It is important for your place of employment to provide a smoke-free environment. If this environment is not presently available, ask to establish an area for smokers that has its own ventilation system.

### *Lewis Harrison's Nine Antidotes for Indoor Pollution are:*

1. Use an electromagnetic shield on your video display terminal to cut low-frequency magnetic field emissions by 98 percent. These shields are available for most computers.
2. Make sure your laser printer has a filter that removes the ozone it produces.
3. Don't buy furniture with foam cushions and upholstery unless the product is made without chlorofluorocarbons, which are used to inflate foam products but which destroy the Earth's protective stratospheric ozone layer.
4. Use furniture made with water-based adhesives and finishes.
5. Choose natural fiber carpeting and upholstery over synthetics, which release volatile organic compounds into the air.
6. Fill your office with plants and flowers. Spider plants and plants with hairy leaves absorb air pollutants (such as formaldehyde), produce oxygen, and add color to ease your eyes. Chrysanthemums, azaleas, and Gerbera daisies are similarly helpful.
7. Ask your cleaning service to use nontoxic, natural cleaners.
8. Typewriter correction fluids contain harmful chemicals that can deplete the stratospheric ozone layer. Try Opti brand, non-toxic correction fluid that won't dry out when the bottle is still half full. It even smells fruity!
9. Implement a no-smoking policy in the office.

How An Executive Got Rid Of Her Headaches By Throwing Out Her Carpet

*Gail T. was a 50-year-old executive who had been complaining for ten years about aggravating and painful headaches. It*

*would start over her left eye and then get worse as her work day passed. The agonizing, throbbing pain was becoming increasingly unbearable. An athlete with healthy eating habits, Gail was baffled by what the cause might be. During a consultation with my staff, it was discovered that she never had these headaches at home. After a few consultations, it was determined that the headaches had begun only when she had moved into her present office. After investigating various factors, Gail obtained some of the same type of foam padding that was under her office carpet. She took some of it home and left it on her work desk. Sure enough she began getting these same headaches at home. When she removed the foam from her presence at home, the headaches ceased. After having sensitivity tests conducted by a holistic doctor, she was told that she was reacting both to the dust in the carpet as well as to the formaldehyde foam. Gail removed the carpet from her office the very next day. In less than a week, her condition had improved so much that it was hard to believe that she had ever had such painful headaches.*

## DO YOU SUFFER FROM SUNLIGHT STARVATION?

All life on our planet has adapted to and is nourished by light from the sun and sky, a critical balance of visible color and invisible ultraviolet wavelengths. Over the ages, virtually every living thing developed with the help of nature's full spectrum.

Today, most people suffer from sunlight starvation because they spend so much time indoors. Get your daily requirements for sunlight! People need sunshine. It's vital to life and health.

## THE MAGIC OF FULL-SPECTRUM LIGHTING

One way to avoid sunlight starvation is through full spectrum indoor lighting. This type of light simulates the full color and beneficial ultraviolet spectrum of sunlight. The full visible and ultraviolet spectrum of natural white light promotes magical healing benefits as no other artificial light can.

### 3 Benefits of Full Spectrum Lighting

1. Students demonstrated increased visual acuity and reduced fatigue while studying under full-spectrum lighting.

2. There was an increased rate of intestinal calcium absorp (necessary for proper bone metabolism), probably due to Vitamin D synthesis.

3. People feel better and experience less of the "winter blues."

People see better under full-spectrum lighting because it reveals detail and color accurately. This type of lighting is a beautiful all-purpose white light — a pleasing, healthful fluorescent tube that operates in existing fixtures for complete lighting of offices, factories, stores, schools, hospitals, banks, or wherever a regular fluorescent light bulb is used.

Look for full-spectrum light bulbs at your local health food store, hardware store, or light fixtures store.

## CLEANING UP OUR WATER

Water is something that many of us take for granted. But it is the magic ingredient to the maintenance of life. There was a time when you could feel secure that the water coming out of your tap was clear and pure and free of undesirable bacteria and contaminants. But those happy days are no longer with us.

Over the last 20 years, hundreds of outbreaks of disease or poisoning caused by contaminated drinking water have been discovered from the Environmental Protection Agency. Water supply experts believe that perhaps ten times as many such incidents occur but go unreported for a variety of reasons. Countless individual sufferers and their doctors may fail to associate ailments with contaminated water.

Although the federal government has set standards for drinking water, many authorities in water treatment have seen these as inadequate at best. Inadequately purified water can contribute to the toxic overload your body must struggle with each day.

### *Six Unhealthy "Additives" You May Be Drinking Every Day*

1. Turbidity
2. Pesticide contamination
3. Fluoridation
4. Industrial pollution
5. Bacterial contamination
6. Chemicals on home, gardens, and lawn
7. Leaching of chemicals from garbage dumps

8. Certain cancer producing chemicals that may be formed by chlorine treatment of drinking water

## MAKING HOME WATER TREATMENT SYSTEMS WORK FOR YOU

People are looking for safer alternatives to tap water. For good health and healing, it is important to use the purest and highest quality water. Many of us use bottled water, but it isn't always easy to know what's in the bottled water we buy.

Although many bottling companies go beyond what the law requires to purify their water, others are not so conscientious. Bacteria can survive the bottling process if the water is not sterilized and can multiply if the bottles stay on the supermarket shelf or in your cupboard for over a month. Unfortunately it is not always possible to determine how long bottled water has been on the shelf since it is not usually labeled with an expiration date.

### 4 Home Water Treatment Systems: The Pros and Cons

1. *Distillation:* Water is vaporized then condensed leaving behind the dissolved minerals.
2. *Deionization of Charcoal Purification:* Water is passed through resins which remove most of the dissolved minerals.
3. *Charcoal Purification:* The most popular water filters on the market today are the small units containing carbon that attach to the end of the faucet. These filters can remove odors, unpleasant tastes, and some murkiness, but they cannot remove bacteria. After a period of use, these charcoal filters have been reported to actually increase the bacterial activity in the water passing through the unit.
4. *Reverse osmosis:* Water is force under pressure though membranes which remove almost all of the dissolved minerals.

Of all the water choices available, I choose the distilled or reversed osmosis variety as the water of choice.

There is no water that is purer than these waters. In distillation the water is boiled and the resultant steam is recondensed. Since rain picks up impurities as it falls through the atmosphere, even rainwater is not as pure as distilled water. Distilled water is probably also the least expensive of the bottled water.

There is an old myth in natural food circles that the use of distilled water for long periods of time may result in the loss of minerals from the body. There is no scientific evidence to support this belief. The respected naturopath Paavo Airola suggested that people concerned about this should remineralize the water by adding bottled sea water for fortification. Distilled water can be made at home with one of the many commercial units that can be purchased from housewares stores or from direct marketing salespeople.

### The Purifying Benefits of Clean Water

1. Cleanses the internal organs
2. Moves nutrients throughout the system
3. Maintains body temperature
4. Helps eliminated toxins form the bloodstream
5. Reduces hunger

HOW MYSTERY ALLERGIES MIRACULOUSLY CLEARED UP BY SWITCHING TO DISTILLED WATER

*Bill P. a 35-year-old man who held an important position in a large mining company in Wales, had been suffering from allergies for several years. Sometimes the fatigue, runny nose, and watery eyes he experienced were so bad that he was confined to bed. The usual remedies (aspirin, antihistamines, and allergy shots) had not helped. That week an article was printed in Bill P.'s local paper celebrating the high quality of the area's drinking water: chlorinated and fluoridated, it was designed to kill bacteria and prevent tooth decay. Bill P. remembered that his allergies became worse whenever he would jog and then drink eight to ten glasses of water. Believing that the water might just be the culprit. I suggested that Bill switch to distilled water; absent of any chemicals, gases, and minerals, was the purest of waters. Within a week, Bill was completely free of his allergy symptoms.*

# HOW TO
# BUILD A
# HEALTHY BODY

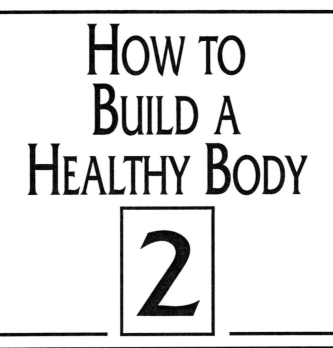

As we have seen in Chapter One, having a healthy body means being free from the effects of artificial additives and toxic environmental situations. Good health means more than just freedom from disease. A truly healthy body will sleep well, awake refreshed, and be confident and capable throughout the day. Good health includes a sense of vitality and the ability to experience pleasure and joy. A healthy body will also be able to experience occasional pain or discomfort without feeling overwhelmed by it.

In short, a healthy body is a happy body. A happy body can be like your best friend—someone you can count on to be there for you through good times and bad, someone who is a pleasure to be with, someone whose company you truly enjoy.

Getting the "junk" out of our lives is a good start on the road to a healthy, happy body. The next step is to put the good stuff back in. To learn to eat what is good for us, most of us need a little bit of guidance, especially at first because we are often unaware or misinformed regarding what our bodies really need to be fed. Reading through the following sections will help to fill in any gaps you may have in your nutritional knowledge, and will also help to dispel some of the many food myths that may have confused you in the past. I will also be showing you health restoring exercises and visualization techniques to help you step up to the next level of health.

## REQUIRED EATING:
## THE SIX ESSENTIAL NUTRIENTS

Among all the nutritional factors that we read about there are six that are considered to be "essential." This means that if you do not get all of them somewhere in your diet, you will cease to live!

These essential nutrients are

1. Protein
2. Fats
3. Carbohydrates
4. Vitamins
5. Minerals
6. Water

Your healthy body must have these nutrients to perform well as you digest your food, fight off disease, use your muscles, repair damaged tissue, and grow healthy new tissue.

For these and hundreds of other daily activities, the six essential nutrients really are not only recommended but absolutely required.

## *Vitamins and Their Sources*

Vitamins are essential body-building elements and play an important role in the prevention of illness. Fresh fruits and vegetables are the best sources of these nutrients, which are destroyed when food is overexposed to air, heat, and light.

| Vitamins | Best Sources | Functions |
|---|---|---|
| Vitamin A | fish, cabbage, carrots, celery, dandelions, spinach, watercress, orange | Aids skin, eyes, liver, bone growth, kidney, muscles, lungs, and heart function. |
| Thiamine ($B_1$) | brewer's yeast, whole grains, wheat germ | Helps build and nurture cells. Breaks down carbohydrates. |

| | | |
|---|---|---|
| Riboflavin (B$_2$) | brewer's yeast, whole grains, wheat germ | Helps carry hydrogen and oxygen through the body |
| Niacin (B$_3$) | brewer's yeast, whole grains, wheat germ | Affects the skin, nerves, digestion, and vision. |
| Pyridoxine (B$_6$) | brewer's yeast, whole grains, wheat germ, potatoes, green, leafy vegetables | Helps build blood cells and control cholesterol, which in excessive amounts can cause a blockage in blood flow and lead to hardening of the arteries. |
| Vitamin B$_{12}$ | Many nutrition books claim that animal proteins are the only sources for this vitamin; however, large amounts can be obtained from micro algae like spirulina and chlorella as well as from dairy products | Essential for normal functioning of all cells, particularly bone marrow, the nervous system, and the digestive system. Needed for red blood cell formation. |
| Biotin | brewer's yeast, wheat germ | Essential in the formation of nucleic acid and glycogen. Is required in the synthesis of several of the nonessential amino acids, which are building blocks of protein. |
| Pantothenic Acid | tomatoes, nuts, potatoes, green vegetables, and molasses | Helps to maintain blood sugar and to resist body stress. |
| Folic Acid | green, leafy vegetables, brewer's yeast | Sparks action from vitamins A, D, E, and K. Also affects the liver, kidneys, and blood. |
| Vitamin C | lemons, oranges, grapefruit, green peppers, tomatoes, berries, rose hips, watercress | Helps form red blood cells, protects and promotes bone and tissue growth, and builds the body's resistance |

|  |  | to disease. Acts as a catalyst to spark action of other vitamins. |
|---|---|---|
| *Vitamin D* | *cod liver oil* | *Helps preserve calcium and phosphorus in the blood. Nourishes the blood.* |
| *Vitamin E* | *green, leafy vegetables, wheat germ, vegetable oils, nuts, whole grains* | *Breaks up cholesterol. Is a healing agent. Increases stamina.* |
| *Vitamin F (Essential fatty acids)* | *pumpkin seeds, sunflower seeds, other nuts* | *Keeps tissues functioning.* |
| *Vitamin K* | *watercress, cabbage and other green vegetables* | *Helps clotting of blood.* |

## *Minerals and Their Sources*

Minerals are the essential building materials of the body and were recognized as essential to human nutrition long before vitamins were discovered. Although vitamins are used by the body in relatively small amounts, many minerals are needed in quantities of one gram or more. Minerals are more important in our diets than many people realize, and most diets are seriously deficient in them. Neither muscles nor nerves can function properly unless they are bathed in tissue fluids that contain certain amounts of mineral salts.

| *Minerals* | *Best Sources* | *Functions* |
|---|---|---|
| *Calcium* | *dairy products, dark-green vegetables, nuts, beans, and seeds* | *Develops bones and teeth. Assists in the movement of muscles and the clotting of blood.* |
| *Chloride* | *kelp and other sea vegetables* | *Though seldom discussed, is part of hydrochloric acid, which is used in digestion.* |

|  |  | Also affects muscle functioning and provides life-sustaining elements. |
|---|---|---|
| Chromium | brewer's yeast | Increases the effectiveness of insulin and stimulates the enzyme involved in glucose metabolism. |
| Cobalt | soybeans | Essential for the formation of vitamin $B_{12}$. |
| Copper | green, leafy vegetables | An essential mineral found in all body tissues, though very little is required. |
| Iodine | kelp, sea vegetables, turnip tops | Was first nutrient considered essential to human beings. Affects the thyroid gland and many metabolic functions of the body. |
| Iron | molasses, green, leafy vegetables, sea vegetables, raisins, apricots | Provides oxygen and helps it to be utilized by the body. |
| Magnesium | soy flour, whole wheat, brown rice, nuts, beans, molasses | Stimulates brain impulses and muscle contractions. Affects the glands. |
| Manganese | bananas, beans, wheat bran, celery, nuts | Is an important catalyst and component of many enzymes in the body. |
| Phosphorus | beans, soy flour, whole wheat | Has more functions than any other mineral, including the formation of strong bones and teeth. |
| Potassium | bananas, oranges, green, leafy vegetables, nuts, beans | Stimulates nerve impulses for muscle contraction. Helps maintain water balance and distribution. |

| | | |
|---|---|---|
| | | *Necessary for healthy functioning of the adrenal glands.* |
| *Selenium* | *brewer's yeast* | *Serves as an anti-oxidant and is believed to be a cancer prevention agent.* |
| *Sodium* | *celery, kelp, and other sea vegetables* | *Works with chloride to regulate the pH balance of body fluids.* |
| *Sulfur* | *wheat germ, beans, cheese, peanuts, garlic* | *Maintains sugar level in the blood. Affects the hair and all cells.* |
| *Zinc* | *pumpkin seeds, beans (especially lentils), peas, spinach* | *Is a component of insulin. Stimulates the enzymes involved in digestion and metabolism.* |

Additional minerals that have a place in nutrition are vanadium, molybdenum, nickel, tin, silicon, aluminum. Minerals that have no known requirement and can be toxic include cadmium, lead, and mercury.

## THE HIGH- PROTEIN MYTH

As important as protein is to good health, Americans have become obsessed with "high-protein" diets. This is a trend that began at the end of World War II and continued into the early 1980s. There was even a point where some nutritionists were recommending an intake as high as 150 grams of protein a day. People had to eat large amounts of red meat to achieve this level. A more commonly accepted view by many researchers is that people can live healthily with a protein intake as low as 30 grams. Though this may be too low a daily protein intake for most people, it is notable in its contrast to the high-protein levels that were recommended by physicians not so long ago. Generally, most healthy people will use approximately 50 to 80 grams of protein per day. In place of all that red meat and animal protein, we now know that combinations of various vegetarian foods are a much healthier choice.

Due to general life-style factors and the history of how we were fed by our parents, many of us believe that beef, chicken, whole milk products, and eggs are the best sources of protein. This belief has changed somewhat as we have learned about reducing our fat intake by cutting back on red meat. Although beef, chicken, whole milk products, and eggs all have plenty of protein, they may also be laden with pesticides, hormones, saturated fats, and various body-polluting substances. Luckily there are many foods that, when eaten alone or in combination with each other, will offer high-quality protein without the fat or undesirable chemicals.

## *Carcinogens Associated with Consumption of Meat*

| *Carcinogen* | *Source* | *Effects* |
|---|---|---|
| Arsenic | Added to hog and poultry feed | Associated with cancer of the liver |
| Benzo(a)pyrene | Charcoal broiling of steaks | Produces stomach cancer and leukemia in laboratory animals; may be transmitted to fetus by pregnant mothers |
| Cancerous tissue | Meat containing cancerous grow tissue which that has been overlooked or inadequately excised | Suspected of carcinogenthesis |
| Diethylstilbestrol (DES) and other hormones | Administered to cattle to promote growth and regulate sexual activity | Produces renal cancer in laboratory mice; associated with vaginal cancer in women whose mothers had been treated with DES |
| Leukemia virus | Meat from poultry and cattle harboring the virus | Suspected of causing human leukemia |
| Malenaldehyde | Oxidation of polyunsaturated fatty acids | Produces cancer in laboratory animals |

| | | |
|---|---|---|
| Methyl-cholanthrene | High-temperature heating of animal fat | Predisposes laboratory animals to cancer; may be transmitted to fetus by pregnant mothers |
| Nitrosamines | Reaction of sodium nitrite in cured meats with urea or amines produced by degradation of protein | Produces various types of cancer in laboratory animals; may be transmitted to fetus by pregnant mothers |
| Pesticides | Ingestion and accumulation in animal tissues through consumption of contaminated forage and grains | Produce liver cancer in laboratory mice |

One of the best ways to obtain high-quality protein without the body-polluting factors is to eat combinations of grains and beans along with some low-fat milk products. The 30 Day Body Purification Program recipe for Soy Burgers (see recipes Appendix VII) is a perfect example of a high-quality protein dish you might prepare for yourself or for your family.

Some people may be allergic or sensitive to all milk products. For these individuals soy milk or goat's milk can serve as an adequate replacement. Experiment with different low-fat milks to see which tastes best to you.

### A Switch to Healthier Proteins Clears Up Respiratory Problems and Eases Arthritis

*Mrs. Loretta H., 57 years old, short in stature, weighing 185 pounds, with high blood pressure, blotchy skin rashes, arthritis pain in both knees, and headaches came to me in agony. Hardly able to walk more than one block and even that, only when supported by a cane, she claimed to be ready, willing, and able to change her dietary habits. I began her purification program by slowly replacing her intake of animal proteins with plant-based proteins. Wanting to avoid a drastic reaction I did not initially eliminate any of her other normal patterns no matter how questionable. My belief was that simply reducing her intake of beef, poultry, eggs, and fish and increasing her use of grain and bean*

*combinations, tofu, tempeh, and low-fat dairy products would
create an immediate shift. This belief was quickly shown to be a
correct one. The dietary change initially brought her weight down
4 pounds a week. Slowly adding juices, more salads, and steamed
vegetables helped normalize her weight loss to a steady level of 2
to 3 pounds per week. To her weight loss and healing, exercise
and meditation were added as well. After four weeks her skin
cleared up, and her condition was so much better that she was
able to walk a mile a day.*

## "GOOD" FATS VERSUS "BAD" FATS

When you talk about body purification, the first negative thing that
often comes to people's minds is fat. This is unfortunate since the proper use of fat in the diet is so important to good health.

Of all the nutrients, fats provide the most concentrated source of
energy. Pound for pound, fat supplies more than twice as much energy
as carbohydrates or protein. Loosely speaking, fats are not one substance. They are actually made up of various fatlike substance known
as lipids. These lipids can include triglyceride, sterols, phospholipids,
fat-soluble vitamins, and tocopherols. The different combinations of
lipids give each fat a unique flavor, melting point, and texture.

Certain fats have properties that make them solid at room temperature. These fats are said to be "saturated." Butter, beef fat, and
cream are considered to have large amounts of saturated fatty acids.
Fats that are liquid at room temperature are called "unsaturated."
These are what we generally call "oils." Most animal fats are saturated;
most fats from vegetable origins are unsaturated, with the exception of
coconut, avocado, and some palm fats. Examples of unsaturated oils
are corn, sunflower, safflower, and sesame oils.

One of the key factors in an effective body purification program
is to get the amount and type of fat that will fulfill the body's requirements while reducing your intake of fats and oils to a healthy level.
This involves issues of both quantity and quality. A diet that is high in
saturated fatty acids has been found to decrease the flow of essential
oxygen to the tissues, creating a condition called anoxia throughout the
body. Therefore, it is important to replace the saturated and chemically processed fats and oils that you may have been using with high-quality expeller pressed oils.

Often certain solid cooking fats and margarines that are made from vegetable rather than animal sources claim to be made from "polyunsaturated oils." These are highly undesirable products that have been saturated by artificial hydrogenation (the adding of hydrogen to created the hardening effect). These are essentially synthetic foods that are questionable at best as a source of fat in a nutritionally balanced diet. At worst, polyunsaturated oils create potential health problems These products also tend to have large amounts of artificial flavors, colors, and preservatives.

In addition to saturated and polyunsaturated fats and oils (fish oils may be one or the other depending on the type of fish), there is a third category of fat classification: monounsaturated fats. These go one step farther. Monounsaturated fats appear to decrease the level of damaging LDL (low-density lipoprotein) cholesterol in the blood, while helping to preserve the level of beneficial HDL (high-density lipoprotein) cholesterol.

Research is showing that the real issue at hand is not simply which is better, saturated or unsaturated fat, but rather the level of essential fatty acids that they contain. There are two essential fatty acids, linoleic acid and linoleic acid.

Although deficiencies of essential fatty acids were thought to be rare, experts are beginning to suggest that the condition may be more widespread than previously thought. Many people who exhibit the following symptoms have been found to have abnormally low blood and/or tissue levels of these essential fatty acids.

> *Insufficient Linoleic Acid:* Behavioral changes, thirst and abnormal water loss through the skin, kidney degeneration, hair loss, arthritis, heart, problems, circulatory problems, poor wound healing, poor growth, miscarriage in females, sterility in males, reduced immunity, eczema-type skin eruptions, gallbladder problems, prostatitis, acne, and muscle tremors.

> *Insufficient Linolenic Acid:* Poor growth, impaired, vision, impaired learning ability, poor motor coordination, and tingling in the legs and arms.

All these symptoms will clear up if adequate amounts of these essential fatty acids (EFAs) are returned to the diet. Good sources of EFAs are canola oil, flaxseed oil, borage oil, walnut oil, and good old monounsaturated olive oil. All these also tend to be very low in saturated fat.

### LOWER CHOLESTEROL LEVELS AND CLEAR UP SKIN RASHES WITH FLAXSEED OIL AND BORAGE OIL

*Bob C., a 35-year-old factory worker, was told by his doctor that he had high cholesterol. He also had been suffering from skin rashes. Repeated treatment by doctors did not bring any permanent relief.*

*In May 1988, he came under my care. Seeing he was moderately obese, I reduced his intake of fatty foods and added flaxseed and borage oil in supplement form and prescribed a reducing cure. After two weeks, not only did his cholesterol began to drop, but his skin rashes started to clear up. After two months his cholesterol was normal and his skin rash was completely gone.*

## COMPLEX CARBOHYDRATES: A NUTRITIONAL GOLD MINE

Carbohydrates are the primary source of energy for your healthy body. Carbohydrates supply energy for muscular exertion, for digestion and absorption of other foods, and for the proper functioning of your brain and nervous system. By furnishing this kind of energy, carbohydrates actually lessen the need of protein intake to perform these tasks. Your body is then free to utilize any protein you consume to repair damaged tissue and to build healthy new tissue.

In trying to reduce your weight to "ideal" levels, carbohydrates have an advantage over fats: carbohydrates contain less than half the number of calories per ounce as fats. Complex carbohydrate foods are better than simple carbohydrate foods in this regard. Simple carbohydrates — such as sugars — provide calories but little else in the way of nutrients.

Carbohydrates, in their complex form, are essential for purification and rejuvenation. In addition to providing energy, many carbohydrate foods supply significant amounts of minerals, B vitamins, and protein. Complex carbohydrates also help detoxify the body by converting certain chemicals, bacterial toxins, and some normal metabolites (the end products of the physical and chemical processes involved in the maintenance of life) into a form that can be easily eliminated as waste.

Complex carbohydrate foods include beans, peas, nuts, seeds, vegetables, and whole grain breads, cereals, and pasta. Starches, the best form of carbohydrates, include whole grains like brown rice, millet, buckwheat (also known as kasha) and barley, along with beans and rootlike vegetables, such as potatoes, carrots, and yams. During the 30-Day Body Purification Program, you will want to add an increasing variety of these cleansing, energy-packed, mineral-rich foods to your daily diet. Be sure to avoid white rice, prepared cereals, and refined white flour products, such as macaroni, bread, and crackers.

## *The Essential Nutrients*

The major nutrient groups are proteins, carbohydrates fats, vitamins, minerals, and water. They are responsible for the following functions:

### *Proteins*
- *Growth and repair body tissue.*
- *Structure of body cells.*
- *Maintenance of normal fluid balance.*
- *Regulation of body functions.*
- *Production of antibodies to fight infection and disease.*

### *Carbohydrates*
- *Main source of energy for all tissues, including the brain and nervous system.*
- *Source of glucose for nerve tissues.*

### *Fats*
- *Concentrated source of energy.*
- *Source of essential fatty acids.*
- *Transportation and absorption by body cells of fat-soluble vitamins. A, D, E, and K.*

### *Vitamins*
- *Maintenance of body processes.*
- *Effective use of other nutrients.*
- *Normal physical and mental development.*

### *Minerals*
- *Building materials for bones, teeth, and other tissues such as blood and nerves.*

- *Regulation of body processes.*
- *Maintenance of normal fluid and acid-base balance.*

*Water*

- *Essential, major constituents of all body cells.*
- *Removal of waste from the body.*

## FIBER: NATURE'S PURIFIER

In recent years, various studies have shown the importance of fiber in reducing the risk of certain types of cancer and heart disease. One type of fiber found in many carbohydrate foods is cellulose. Although it is essentially indigestible by humans, cellulose is one of the key sources of fiber that your body requires for healthy digestion and elimination. You can increase the amount of cellulose in your diet by eating more complex carbohydrate foods and by not peeling all your fruits and vegetables. A well-scrubbed apple/carrot/potato peel a day, whether cooked, juiced or steamed, or raw, will really keep that doctor away!

CURE CONSTIPATION AND HEMORRHOIDS BY INCREASING DIETARY FIBER

*In the summer of 1990, Betty M., a 52-year-old owner of a fast-food, restaurant came to my office in a desperate mood. She had not moved her bowels in over 5 days. The usual treatment—laxatives applied for five weeks—had not helped. She was suffering from abdominal cramps and painful hemorrhoids. I recommended oat meal and oat bran for breakfast, beans soups, salads with 2 tablespoons of olive oil, and eight glasses of water daily. I also restricted her intake of refined foods, especially pasta, white bread, and white rice. The problem cleared up as well as her hemorrhoidal pain, and she returned to work.*

## THE HEALING POWER
## OF MOVEMENT

A proper fitness program can improve every aspect of your life! It can increase your energy and improve your mental and physical capabilities, while at the same time expanding your alertness. It can also do wonders for your emotional health.

Regular exercise helps prevent heart attacks, aids in weight control by increasing your metabolism, instills a feeling of well-being, and helps people troubled by diabetes, ulcers, nervous tension, high blood pressure, back pain, recurrent headaches, menstrual cramps, hangovers, constipation, and insomnia.

In study after study, scientists have shown that exercise improves moods and emotional health. The latest studies from Stanford University reveal that endorphins, which are morphine like hormones, are released into the brain by vigorous exercise. That is how scientists explain the "high" people often experience after exercising.

According to fitness authority, Dr. Kenneth Cooper, the most popular forms of exercise include brisk walking, hiking, jogging, running, cross-country skiing, swimming, cycling, jumping rope, and studio aerobics.

Although cardiovascular exercise is a must if you want to be at your best, high-impact aerobics (long periods of intense jumping and bobbing) is being replaced by equally effective but easier and less physically damaging low-impact aerobics, in which one foot always remains on the floor.

Low-impact aerobics will make the heart muscle work harder. As with any muscle, the heart will grow stronger the more it is exercised. A strong heart will pump more blood with less effort. New capillaries are formed, thus expanding your body's ability to digest, absorb, and transport oxygen and nutrients to all of your cells and to carry away toxins and wastes to your organs of elimination. Aerobic exercise improves circulation to the largest organ of elimination, your skin, enabling your body to eliminate toxins even more effectively. When combined with good nutrition, aerobic exercise will strengthen the skin's connective tissue and increase its elasticity. Aerobics will cause you to breathe more intensely, giving you a stronger diaphragm and your lungs more elasticity. Low-impact aerobics are also the most efficient way to use up stored fat in the body — and calories continue to be burned at a greater pace for several hours after you have exercised. In the long run, your metabolic rate will increase overall as well! This means that continuing to exercise regularly after losing unwanted weight will help keep those extra pounds from even thinking about settling in again.

Making exercise a priority is important. It is also important to set goals — just make them realistic ones. Don't expect too much too soon. Remember that you may feel a bit worse before you feel better. The key is to have a regular routine and be consistent, and, while you are at it, remember that exercise can be fun! Keep trying different activities until you find a way of exercising that you truly enjoy.

The simplest and most balanced exercises to do during the first three weeks of your program include elements of stretching, vascular training (aerobics), and a focusing or meditative exercise program. These exercises will help you to facility body purification and will give you a variety of exercises to choose from later on. During the fourth week and in the maintenance program that follows the initial 30 days, you will be adding strength training as you learn to build your brand new, healthy body.

Modern life often requires enormous energy and great intensity of mind and body. As you go through your daily activities, lactic acid is formed in the muscle fibers of your body and you become tired and fatigued.

A meditative approach to exercise can ease this aspect of modern living. Practicing proper breathing, a positive mental attitude, concentration, proper warm-up and visualization, less lactic acid will be produced, and you will experience less muscle fatigue and tiredness.

When using exercise as a form of meditation, muscles respond by staying relaxed longer. Many people report that this type of exercise enhances their creativity, Swami Vishnudevananda, a respected yoga teacher, has this to say about the meditative element of yoga and exercise: "Just as water flows through an open tap, so energy flows into the relaxed muscles."

I have interspersed these health-giving exercises with other features and ingredients of the 30-Day Body Purification Program. Incorporate them into your daily routine to experience renewed vitality and well-being.

A MARATHON RUNNER HEALS HER BACKACHES

*Susan P. was a long distance runner who used my exercise and massage program to cure her backaches. Here is how she describes her ordeal:*

*"I've always considered myself to be in great physical condition. I run about forty miles a week, rain or shine, and have done so for years. About two years ago, I began to experience pains in my lower back. It became unbearable. I began using pain killers*

*even though I try to avoid using medication whenever possible. Nothing seemed to help and I was afraid that I might never run again. Sometimes ice packs would help and sometimes hot packs would help. I even tried race walking in the hope that it would put less stress on my back. I went to doctors who X-rayed my spine but they found nothing wrong. I went home disheartened by the situation which got worse. Later the pain would actually start while I was asleep and awaken me. I tried chiropractors, physical therapists, orthopedic doctors. No one was able to isolate the cause or eliminate the pain."*

*When Susan came to me I introduced her to a three part program.*

1. *She began to workout in the gym and signed up for muscle strengthening classes. By strengthening her abdominal muscles, Susan was able to reduce the stress on her lower back muscles.*

2. *She took yoga stretching classes. Although Susan was aerobically fit, her muscles, were out of balance. Her leg muscles were strong but her upper body and back were weak.*

3. *Weekly deep muscle massage. These massages helped reduce stress and tension around the joints and reduced the tightness in the hamstring muscles in the back of Susan's legs.*

*This combination of strengthening, stretching and massage helped eliminate Susan's back pain and she was soon running again.*

### Four Signs That You Have a Healthy Body

1. You wake up feeling rested after a full night's sleep.
2. You are able to easily digest your food.
3. You have full, easy bowel movements.
4. At the end of the day you have a sense of emotional gratification without feeling exhausted.

# WEEK #1 BALANCING YOUR BODY

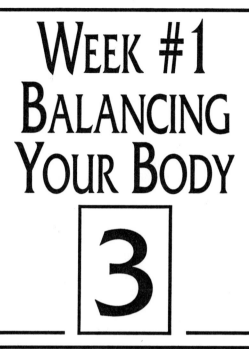

Welcome to Week #1 of Lewis Harrison's 30-Day Body Purification Program! You are about to embark on a journey of discovery of how easy it can be to treat your body in a healthy way. Your body will reward you by becoming cleaner, stronger, and more alive — you will feel the difference! Along the way, you'll gain valuable and up-to-date knowledge about nutrition and healing that can be a help to you and to your loved ones for the rest of your life.

Skip ahead to the grocery list for each week, and then gradually read the information in each chapter throughout that week. Or read each entire chapter from start to finish. With this latter approach, you will know and understand the ideas behind the dietary and exercise changes you are making. Either approach will work — above all, make the program work for you!

There are many things that you can focus on in the application of the 30-Day program. But there are ten key points which if followed consistently will enable you to reap the benefits fully. These are:

# THE TEN COMMANDMENTS OF BODY PURIFICATION

1. Eat a variety of fresh, unrefined, and unprocessed foods.
2. Avoid fat and fatty foods.
3. Eat slowly while sitting down.
4. Choose foods high in complex carbohydrates and high-quality fiber (such as whole grains and beans).
5. Avoid refined white and brown sugar and foods that contain them.
6. If you use sweeteners like honey and maple syrup, do so in moderation.
7. Read labels. Beware of foods that contain artificial colors and flavors, preservatives or high amounts of sodium.
8. Avoid all alcoholic beverages.
9. Avoid caffeine (coffee, iced tea, cola, and nonherbal teas).
10. Exercise (your body *and* your imagination!).

Following these "commandments" is an easy way to bring your body back into the healthy, balanced state it is meant to be in. You will find yourself feeling lighter, cleaner, and more energized with each day on the program. You may even notice that you are feeling more "balanced" emotionally as well. A person with a healthy, thriving, happy body is less likely to be bothered by the obstacles and annoyances we encounter as we go about our day. Remember to look for small shifts in how you are feeling both physically and emotionally — you may be pleasantly surprised!

Whenever possible, purchase fruits, vegetables, nuts, seeds, grains, and beans that have been grown without the use of pesticides and commercial fertilizer. These "pure" foods are commonly called "organically grown."

Look for organically grown produce at health food stores and farmers' markets in your area. There may also be a supermarket filled with wholesome, organically grown foods opening up soon in your neighborhood. This is an encouraging part of the recent trend toward healthier living in general — support your local organic grocery, or if there isn't one near you, start asking your regular grocer to provide organically grown produce as an alternative.

If it is not practical or possible to obtain organically grown foods right away, it is still possible to use simple, unprocessed foods in all your meal plans. Unprocessed foods will help your body detoxify and grow healthy.

### Six Foods for All Seasons

1. Fresh fruits (raw or cooked)
2. Fresh vegetables (raw or steamed)
3. Whole grain breads, cereals, pastas, and so on
4. Yogurt, buttermilk, unprocessed cheeses, and other low-fat milk products
5. Dry beans and peas
6. Sprouts

Because animal products (meat, fish, poultry, and dairy products) are sources of complete protein, it was thought for many years that they were also the best protein sources. In recent years, however, people have learned that though most vegetable products are not complete proteins, they can be eaten with other vegetable products that contain the complementary amino acids. There are many enjoyable and tasty combinations of nonanimal foods that create perfectly nutritious and balanced protein. These "complete" protein combinations also lack the negative aspects of certain animal foods. Pesticide residues, undesirable chemical additives, and hormones used in the production of poultry create problems similar to those associated with beef.

As you begin to shift your diet to include new types of high-quality protein, decrease your intake of meats and high-fat dairy products. Foods that are rich in complex carbohydrates are often good sources of protein as well. They are less costly foods and are good sources of vitamins and minerals too. You'll also benefit from a lower intake of saturated fats and cholesterol.

If you feel that you have to have some animal protein in your diet, then eat organically grown poultry and lamb or veal instead of beef or pork. If you are ready to make a greater adjustment to your diet, consider using non-fat milk products and grain and bean combinations as your primary protein sources.

Try these sources of high-quality protein throughout the first seven days of your program:

A lactovegetarian diet using only dairy products that are pre-pared from part skim or nonfat milk.

Low-fat or dry curd cottage cheese instead of creamed cottage cheese.

Nonfat dry milk powder for quiches and custards to prevent a watery texture.

Tempeh.

Tofu.

Brewer's yeast, primary grown yeast, and nutritional yeast. All these yeasts are available in tablet or powder form and are extremely economical. They vary in taste from brand to brand but can be very pleasant to use, once you find a brand that you like.

Micro algae. The nutritional content of these little green plants is very high, especially the protein and chlorophyll content. The most popular of the microalgaes are chlorella and spirulina.

### Purifying Protein Combos

Red or black beans and brown rice

Split pea soup and whole grain bread sticks

Corn and bean salad

Black-eyed peas and corn bread

Whole wheat bread and unsweetened natural peanut butter

Whole corn tortillas and refried beans

Whole wheat bread baked with soy flour in the dough mixture

Bean soup (pea, lentil, lima bean, and so on) with sesame seeds or sunflower seeds added

HOW SEA VEGETABLES HELP STIMULATE A SLUGGISH THYROID AND RELIEVE CONSTIPATION

*Sara was the secretary of a very high-ranking and internation-ally known statesman and member of the Spanish royal family. She was a 41-year-old woman whose brown hair had turned white at the age of 36. I knew that this often indicates glandular or meta-bolic disturbances. She had been suffering for several years from a mild but chronic thyroid condition, which caused her to gain weight and feel sluggish all the time. In connection with this con-*

*dition, she had also experienced periodic episodes of constipation. She sometimes experienced terrible flushes, after which she would be dripping wet from sweat, also experiencing the sensation of palpitations in her heart. All the usual treatments did not help. By adding plenty of sea vegetables to her diet (nori, hijiki, dulse, kombu, wakame), she lost weight, gained energy, and obtained regular bowel movements, making her completely free from distress within two months.*

## REPLACING BAD FATS WITH GOOD FATS

One of the most important elements of an effective body purification program is the replacement of saturated and chemically processed fats and oils with high-quality expeller pressed oils.

Over the years, studies have shown that even polyunsaturated fats advertised so aggressively on television have certain qualities to question. For example reports have indicated that large quantities of vegetable oil in the diet speed up the aging process in the skin, with the result of increased wrinkling about the face. According to Nathan Pritikin, the developer of the famous Pritikin Diet, all fats, including animal and vegetable, have the common effect of causing red blood cells and platelets and other elements in the blood to stick together. One of the results of this clumping is that capillaries and other small blood vessels become clogged and shut down. A good part of the problem with oils can be traced to the highly reactive oxygen that they carry. The heating of oils (and the most natural of oils involves heat in the extraction process) speeds up the oxidation process, resulting in earlier rancidity. Many healers feel that using any processed oil, no matter how natural, is to be avoided. This becomes a difficult issue for many nutritionists in light of the therapeutic benefits that have been associated with olive oil and recent research praising cod liver and other fish oils. Since natural oils contain certain antioxidants and natural preservatives, such as vitamin E, lecithin, and sesamol (an unrefined sesame oil), these may be safe to use within a short time of purchase if used in moderation. It is important to remember that vegetable oils typically purchased in supermarkets have been extensively processed (refined, deodorized, and bleached) and have less nutritional value and no therapeutic value when compared to "cold pressed," "expeller pressed," and other naturally prepared oils.

When you purchase a naturally processed oil, be sure that it comes in a dark bottle and keep it refrigerated. You should not keep it in storage for more than a month or so, and, if you wish, you can even put a few drops of Vitamin E liquid into the bottle to reduce the potential for spoilage. Avoid cooking, frying, or broiling with oils whenever possible.

Fats that have large amounts of saturated fatty acids include.

> Butter
> Beef fat
> Milk fat (cream)

Examples of unsaturated liquid fats (oils) are.

> Corn
> Sunflower
> Safflower
> Sesame oil

To increase good fats and oils and reduce bad ones:

- Choose dry beans and peas (in combination with whole grains) as protein sources, rather than beef, pork, and whole milk products.
- When using milk products, use skim or low-fat milk products.
- Limit your intake of eggs and poultry.
- Limit your intake of fats and oils, especially foods high in saturated fat, for example, butter, cream, lard, heavily hydrogenated fats (this includes many margarines), shortenings, and foods containing palm and/or coconut oils.
- When using oil in dressings or in food preparation, always choose canola oil or extra-virgin olive oil that has been cold pressed.
- Avoid foods that have been fried. Broil, bake, or steam your food whenever possible. Steaming is superior to boiling because there is less nutrient loss that way.

### Four Super Healing Oils to Try

*Sesame:* Wonderful with whole grains, noodles and oriental dishes.

*Olive:* The oil of choice for salads and sauces. The best olive oil to use is unfiltered extra virgin.

*Sunflower:* A mild-tasting oil with a high nutrition value. It can be used when you wish to lighten the fuller taste of olive oil.

*Canola:* High in monounsaturates and the Omega-3 fatty acids associated most often with fish oils.

## THE HEALING POWER OF FERMENTED MILK PRODUCTS

It is generally believed that fermented milk products such as yogurt, buttermilk, and kefir have been used as food for over 6,000 years. Legend states that a merchant traveling in Mesopotamia carried some milk in a sack made from the stomach of a sheep. He expected to find cool milk, but, at the end of the day, he found a thick, creamy, slightly sour milk product. Apparently, bacteria from the bag, heated by the sun, had combined with the milk; when the temperature dropped suddenly at night, the milk curdled and bacterial action stopped. The camel driver found that, by mixing the creamy curd with water, he could drink it with greater ease and that it was extremely thirst quenching. The discovery was passed among nomads who found they could actually create the liquid food by inoculating fresh milk with previously fermented milk.

In 1908, the Russian scientist Metchnikoff wrote that yogurt was the "elixir of life." He advanced the theory that yogurt could counteract the "putrefactive bacteria" in the large intestine that caused disease and shortened life. Metchnikoff reasoned that people in the Caucasus area around the Black Sea lived such long and healthy lives because of the great amount of lactobacillus they ate in their food.

In 1986, the British nutritionist K.W. Heaton reported in the *Journal of the Royal Society of Medicine*, on the Asian people from Gujarat. When these Indians, primarily of the Hindu faith, emigrated to London, they were found to have developed various nutritional problems. These people had traditionally eaten kefir, a yogurtlike food fermented by lactobacillus. Heaton also noted that, in India, people eat imperfectly washed vegetables that are probably covered with lactobacillus from the soil in their gardens. After they moved to

England, they ate well-washed British vegetables purchased from the supermarket. As time passed, and the Indians absorbed traditionally English dietary habits, they began eating an "endless variety of sugary foods and drinks," stopped making kefir, and over a few years, began to "manifest a high prevalence of obesity, diabetes and coronary heart disease."

Yogurt has been recognized for centuries as having health and dietary benefits, but most manufacturers have taken the cheap route and any great healing benefits to be found in many brands were long since processed out back at the factory. Yogurt, in its most basic form, should contain milk and yogurt culture. Beware of products labeled "natural" that actually contain many additives.

### Six Body-Purifying Fermented Milk Products

1. *Whole Milk Yogurt:* Because they contain about 4 percent butterfat, these products are richer and thicker than low-fat varieties and do not require any added thickeners.

2. *Low-Fat Yogurts:* These yogurts have less butterfat (1 to 1.5 percent fat). If you are concerned about your weight, the difference between whole milk and skim milk varieties is about 30 calories per 8oz. container of unflavored yogurt. When preserves or flavorings are added, the caloric content per cup of plain skim milk yogurt can increase from about 150 calories to some 250 or more.

3. *Goat Yogurt:* Despite a slightly gamey taste this is a great choice for those who wish to avoid cow's milk.

4. *Kefir:* Kefir is the cultured milk drink that virtually all "yogurt drinks" have attempted to copy. Similar to yogurt in taste and nutritional value, kefir in its original form was prepared from mares' milk by nomads in Asia and Russia who drank it as an alcoholic beverage. Commercially available kefir is alcohol free and is flavored much like yogurt with fruit preserves and sugar. Because there is no purpose in making kefir thick like yogurt, kefir tends to have few or no added artificial ingredients. Kefir is spoonable, like yogurt, but less thick. Most varieties made from low-fat milk have about 85 calories in a 6-oz. serving of plain and 115 calories of fruited. Kefir, then, has the same virtues as any other dairy product: high-quality protein, calcium, and many of the B vitamins. And like yogurt, it can

be made from low-fat milk.

5. *Buttermilk:* Many people believe the myth that butte......... is high in butter due to its name. The truth is that buttermilk is a wonderfully healing food! It is low in fat, high in protein, and high in calcium. Its rich lactic acid content is also healing to the intestines.

6. *Soy or Seed Yogurt:* This is a nondairy product prepared from soy milk or a combination of seeds and acidophilus. It is generally very sour and is popular primarily with people who want to avoid milk products while receiving the benefits of acidophilus.

HOW BUTTERMILK AND YOGURT MADE A BURNED OUT TEACHER FEEL STRONG AGAIN

*From my recent experience, I may also mention the following significant case. Jeff W., a 56-year-old man, had been suffering for four months from fatigue, burnout, and abdominal gas. The family doctor and a noted specialist prescribed digestive aids and an increase in meat (animal protein). This brought no relief during the four months. I recommended the use of high-"acidophilus" foods, including yogurt and buttermilk. Studies show that acidophilus can help build the immune system and restore a toxic colon within 30 days. The high quality protein in these high "acidophilus," low-fat dairy products helped Jeff regain his strength.*

## HEALTHY HOME COOKING: HOW TO MAKE YOUR OWN STEAMER

Steaming vegetables is an important part of the purification program. Steaming enables you to lightly cook vegetables without the use of oil or butter, and, since most vegetables contain plenty of natural sodium, steamed vegetables require very little added salt. No kitchen should be without a steamer.

The bamboo steamer is a wonderful cooking tool that can be found in many oriental food supply stores. Another type is a collapsible stainless steel steamer. If you choose a multilevel-style steamer, remember that food will cook faster in the bottom level. Be sure to rotate the layers or put foods that take longer to cook in that bottom level.

If you prefer to make your own home steamer, follow the instructions given here. You will need one large cookpot, a tin can, and a metal rack.

1. Place a metal rack on top of a can that is approximately three inches high and four inches in diameter.
2. Put this arrangement in a pot with a tight-fitting lid.
3. Pour in distilled water to about one and one-half inches below the rack.
4. Place vegetables on the rack and bring the water to a boil.
5. Reduce the heat once the steam begins to appear.
6. Keep the lid on tightly until the vegetables are tender, but crisp.

CAUTION: *Remember that steam can burn, so tilt the lid away from you as you remove it. Don't allow the water level to drop too low or you may burn the pot and wind up with burned-tasting vegetables.*

### STRENGTHEN A WEAK DIGESTION WITH JUICES AND LIGHTLY STEAMED FOODS

*Ina V., a 46-year-old thin, light-haired woman, had been suffering from repeated attacks of colic, gallstones, and nausea. She had tried many different dietary plans. A program of X-rays and diathermy applied over many months but did not help. I recommended fresh vegetable juices with plenty of cabbage and steamed carrots, yellow and green squash, and sweet potatoes. She also drank large quantities of ginger tea. In a few weeks her condition greatly improved.*

The Body purification Triangle on the next page will show you that Effective Body Purification requires a focus on fresh fruits, vegetables, and whole grains. The less oil and animal derived protein that is used the more effective the program becomes.

### WEEK 1 DAILY MENU PLANS AND EXERCISES
*Menu Plan*

**Day 1**

Breakfast                         *16 oz. Juice formula #1\**
                                  *1/2 cup oatmeal*

---

*Recipes for Stirred beverages, main dishes, soups , and sauces may be found in Appendix IV, "Herbs and Spices," Appendix V, "Your Home Guide to Juicing, and Purification Recipes" Appendix VII, "

*8 oz. nonfat yogurt (plain or flavored)*
*Herbal tea or coffee substitute*

Lunch

*6 oz. Pine Nut Tabbouleh\**
*3/4 cup steamed azuash*
*1 cup of a steamed pleasant-tasting sea veg-*
*    etable*
*(arame, wakamae, kombu, hijiki, nori)*
*1 medium tomato, sliced*
*1 cup romaine lettuce (choice of Spa*
*    Dressing\*)*
*Tofu Raspberry Pudding\**
*Herbal tea or coffee substitute*

Dinner

*6 oz. Millet-Onion Saute\**
*1/2 cup steamed green peas*
*1 cup steamed cauliflower with Tomato*
*    Sauce\**
*1 cup romaine lettuce*
*1 6-oz. serving baked peaches*
*Herbal or coffee substitute*

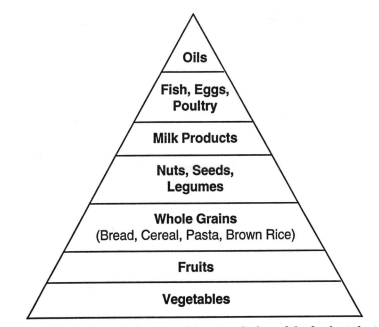

*Use more of the foods at the bottom of the triangle, less of the foods at the top.*

While on the 30 - Day Body Purification Program, you will be putting your body through quite a few changes in diet, cooking habits, even in how you think and feel about food. Learning to relax and allowing these changes to sink in, to become part of your life-style, is an important element of any healing program. Being able to visualize or imagine yourself becoming healthier and more balanced can be very helpful as well.

There are several visualization techniques in the 30-Day Program for you to try. If you find that you enjoy a particular visualization technique, feel free to use it at any time on any day of your program.

## Visualization Technique: Body Purification

Step 1. Find a quiet place where you will not be disturbed.

Step 2. Sit in a straight-backed chair, with both feet flat on the floor and your hands facing palms up and resting on your knees.

Step 3. Close your eyes and inhale and exhale long and slowly.

Step 4. As you exhale, visualize that dust, toxins, and the color gray is leaving your body.

Step 5. Finish this visualization by taking a long deep breath, slowly exhaling, and gradually opening your eyes. Remain quiet for a few minutes while becoming aware of your surroundings without getting up or moving around.

Step 6. Slowly begin to wiggle your toes and fingers.

Step 7. When you feel acclimated to the surrounding environment, you can arise.

*Menu Plan*

**Day 2**

Breakfast            *Citrus Splash Blended Cocktail\**
                     *1/2 cup nonfat, fruit juice-sweeted granola*
                     *Herbal tea or coffee substitute*

Lunch                *6-oz. Mock Chicken Salad\**
                     *3/4 cup steamed white potatoes*
                     *1 medium tomato, sliced*
                     *2 cups romaine lettuce (Choice of*

*Spa Dressing)*
*1 medium apple*
*Herbal tea or coffee substitute*

Dinner

*6 oz. Spicy Mushroom-Sage Stuffing\**
*1 cup of a steamed, pleasant-tasting sea vegetable*
*(arame, wakamae, kombu, hijiki, nori)*
*2 cups romaine lettuce*
*8 oz. nonfat yogurt (plain or flavored)*
*Choice of beverage*

## Contraction-Relaxation Exercises

As your body becomes healthier by being more nutritionally balanced, it is important to become aware of areas of muscular tension and to begin learning to release this tension in a healthy way. These exercises of contracting tense muscles as tight as you can, then releasing the contraction and letting go will help you to achieve a more relaxed state. These exercises are excellent for increasing your energy levels and reducing fatigue.

## Contraction-Relaxation (The Feet and Legs)

Start from your toes and think of each part of the body until you reach your head.

1. Lie down on your back.
2. Bring your attention to the toes in your right foot.
3. Wiggle and stretch them. Spread toes apart. Relax.
4. Bring your attention to your ankle.
5. Rotate your ankle.
6. Flex your calf muscles. Relax.
7. Bring your awareness to your thigh. Tighten it, then more.
8. Lift the straightened leg off the floor 2 inches, tighten more, and then drop it slowly. Relax.
9. Roll your right leg back and forth. Become aware of your left toes. Repeat technique steps 2–8 for your left leg.

*Menu Plan*

**Day 3**

| | |
|---|---|
| Breakfast | *16 oz. Juice Formula #1\** |
| | *1/2 cup nonfat, fruit juice-sweetened granola* |
| | *Herbal tea or coffee substitute* |
| Lunch | *6 oz. Herbed Tofu Pilaf\** |
| | *1 cup chopped cucumber* |
| | *1 medium tomato, sliced* |
| | *1 cup romaine lettuce* |
| | *1 cup of a steamed, pleasant-tasting sea veg-etable* |
| | *(arame, wakamae, kombu, hijiki, nori)* |
| | *1 medium apple* |
| | *Herbal tea or coffee substitute* |
| Dinner | *2 Stuffed Peppers with Basic Mexican Sauce\** |
| | *1/2 cup steamed carrots* |
| | *1 cup steamed carrots* |
| | *1 cup romaine lettuce (choice of Spa Dressing\*)* |
| | *8 oz. nonfat yogurt (plain or flavored)* |
| | *Choice of beverage* |

## Contraction-Relaxation (The Shoulders and Face)

1. Lie down on your back.
2. Bring your attention to your chest and shoulders.
3. Try to make your shoulders touch over chest (this is only an attempt, obviously — they will never reach).
4. Hold for one breath; exhale and drop your shoulders.
5. Bring your attention to your face.
6. Move the muscles in your face, every which way. Make ugly faces and big phony smiles. This will break down the tension.
7. Inhale, then exhale, while releasing contractions in face.
8. Inhale long and deep into your belly. Do not contract muscles. Imagine a stream of white light coming in through your

toes and going out the top of your head. As you imagine this light stream, be aware of the different parts of your body the light stream passes on its journey up and out the top of your head.

*Menu Plan*

**Day 4**

Breakfast

*16 oz. Juice Formula #2\**
*1/2 cup puffed brown rice or millet*
*Herbal tea or coffee substitute*

Lunch

*6 oz. Tempeh Salad\**
*1 cup of a steamed, pleasant-tasting sea vegetable*
*(arame, wakamae, kombu, hijiki, nori)*
*1 cup chopped cucumber*
*1 cup romaine lettuce (choice of Spa Dressing\*)*
*8 oz. nonfat yogurt (plain or flavored)*
*Herbal tea or coffee substitute*

Dinner

*6 oz. Mexican Vegetable Casserole\**
*1/2 cup steamed broccoli*
*1/2 cup steamed cauliflower*
*2 cups romaine lettuce*
*1 serving baked peaches*
*Choice of beverage*

## Body Twist

Based on the Chinese exercise system of T'ai Chi, this technique increases flexibility in the ankles, knees, thighs, and pelvis.

1. Stand with your feet parallel, slightly wider than shoulders, with your knees slightly bent and your hands on your hips.
2. Slowly turn to the right, moving your hips and shoulders perpendicular to feet.
3. Continue turning your head to the right until it is facing 180 degrees from toes.
4. Turn your head to the left, facing same direction as your feet.

5. Turn head same direction as shoulders and hips — and turn all together toward original position.

6. Do steps 2 through 5 on the left side.

Practice this exercise three times on each side; add one cycle a week until you are doing six. Twisting becomes more difficult. The more your knees are bent, the greater the difficulty of the exercise. Be sure to tuck your pelvis slightly forward. Focus your breathing into the center of your belly.

*Menu Plan*

*Day 5*

Breakfast                    *Tropical Quencher Blended Cocktail\**
                             *4 oz. nonfat yogurt with a fresh banana*
                             *Herbal tea or coffee substitute*

Lunch                        *6 oz. Pasta Verde\**
                             *3/4 cup steamed green peas*
                             *1 cup chopped cucumber*
                             *1 cup of a steamed, pleasant-tasting sea veg-*
                             *   etable*
                             *   (arame, wakamae, kombu, hijiki, nori)*
                             *2 cups romaine lettuce (choice of Spa*
                             *   Dressing\*)*
                             *1 medium apple*
                             *Herbal tea or coffee substitute*

Dinner                       *2 Soy Burgers with Homemade Ketchup\**
                             *1/2 cup steamed kale*
                             *1 cup steamed cauliflower*
                             *1 cup romaine lettuce*
                             *Tofu Protein Pops\**
                             *Choices of beverage*

## Abdominal Toner

This exercise is great for toning the abdomen, hips, and back muscles; it also reduces abdominal fat. This exercise comes to us from Kundalini yoga.

1. Place yourself in a sitting position.

2. Extend your legs forward and lean back on your elbows.

3. Lift legs to 60 degrees from floor.
4. While focusing your eyes on your big toes, do the Fire Breath.
5. Exhale and lower your legs.

Start with 15 Fire Breaths. Add 5 each week until you reach 30 breaths. (See Day 19 for a description of Fire Breath)

*Menu Plan*

**Day 6**

Breakfast
*16 oz. Juice Formula #2\**
*1/2 cup oatmeal*
*Herbal tea of coffee substitute*

Lunch
*6 oz. Curried Rice\**
*3/4 cup steamed yellow or zucchini squash*
*    with Chinese Sweet Mustard Sauce\**
*1 cup chopped cucumber*
*1 medium tomato, sliced*
*2 cups romaine lettuce (choice of Spa*
*    Dressing\*)*
*1 medium apple*
*Herbal tea or coffee substitute*

Dinner
*6 oz. Parsley Pasta\**
*1 cup steamed watercress with fresh lemon*
*    juice*
*1 cup romaine lettuce*
*1 cup of a steamed, pleasant-tasting sea veg-*
*    etable*
*    (arame, wakamae, kombu, hijiki, nori)*
*8 oz. nonfat yogurt (plain or flavored)*
*1/2 cup fresh grapes*
*Choice of beverage*

HOW JOSE H. USED NUTRITION TO COMBAT MENTAL AND EMOTIONAL PROBLEMS

*"I was constantly going through mood swings."* This is a 28-year-old man Jose H. describing his mental torture. *"I was always lethargic and depressed. I would lie in bed all day with the*

*covers over my head. My family Doctor said I was schizophrenic but no one knew how to help me and I didn't know how to help myself."*

*Someone called me about Jose and I recommended he see a physician friend of mind who specialized in a holistic approach to emotional and mental problems. After extensive allergy testing, Jose learned that he suffered from low blood sugar (hypoglycemia) as well as a sensitivity to gluten (a protein found in various grains). His low blood sugar was corrected with a thirty day menu described within. He also began to eat small meals in between his three larger main meals. He increased his consumption of beans and seeds. This helped stabilize his sugar levels and his moods became even and less erratic.*

*His physician explained that wheat, rye, barley, malt, and oats are high in gluten and that certain groups of schizophrenics react negatively to gluten.*

*Within thirty days of starting the nutrition program Jose's symptoms began to clear up. His attitude improved, he had more energy and he went into counseling to help him learn to adjust to his new happier emotional state.*

## Back Release

This easy motion helps relieve pelvic and lower back tension.

1. Sit straight in a comfortable chair.
2. While inhaling move your shoulders back, bring your chest up, and move the small of your back forward in one movement.
3. Exhale, pushing back from the small of your back and allowing your chest to drop.

*Menu Plan*

### Day 7

Breakfast

*Sunspice Smoothie Blended Cocktail\**
*8 oz. nonfat yogurt (plain or flavored)*
*Herbal tea or coffee substitute*

Lunch

*6 oz. Pine Nut Tabbouleh\**
*1 cup of a steamed, pleasant-tasting sea vegetable*

*(arame, wakamae, kombu, hijiki, nori)*
*1 cup chopped cucumber*
*1 medium tomato, sliced*
*1 cup romaine lettuce*
*1 medium pear*
*Herbal tea or coffee substitute*

Dinner

*2 Barley Burgers with Basic Mushroom*
   *Sauce\**
*1 whole corn on the cob*
*1 cup steamed cauliflower*
*2 cups romaine lettuce (choice of Spa*
   *Dressing\*)*
*1 serving baked peaches*
*Choices of beverage*

## Forward Stretch

A yoga posture known for stimulating the kidneys, pancreas, and liver; excellent for diabetic patients.

1. Sitting on the floor, extend your legs together in front of you.
2. While inhaling, stretch your arms and torso toward the sky.
3. While exhaling, bend forward, holding onto the first part of your leg that your hands make contact with (This will be somewhere between your foot and knee.)
4. Relax your head and shoulders, close your eyes, and breathe long and deep five breaths.
5. Inhale while you come up slowly and lie on your back.
6. Take 5 long, deep breaths and repeat the cycle. Add 5 cycles each week until you reach 15 cycles.

Remember: Keep legs straight, back of knees on the floor.

## SUGGESTED GROCERY LIST FOR WEEK 1

*Fresh Vegetables:* Squash, Tomatoes, Romaine Lettuce (About 20 Cups), Green Peas, Cauliflower, White Potatoes, Cucumbers, Carrots, Broccoli, Kale (1/2 Cup), Watercress,

Corn on the Cob (One Ear), Green Peppers, Scallions,
Mushrooms, Celery, Radishes, Onion, Shallots, Boston Lettuce
(For Selected Recipes If Desired), Beets
*Fresh Fruit:* Apples, Lemons, Grapes (1/4cup), Pear, Bananas,
Pineapple, Peaches (and/or Nectarines)
*Spices:* Pepper (Black and White), Cinnamon, Mint Leaves or
Flakes, Curry Powder, Curry Powder, Dried Thyme, Cayenne
Powder, Dried Basil, Dried Oregano, Dried Rosemary, Bay
Leaves, Chili Powder, Cumin, Coriander, Dry Mustard, Onion
Powder, Sea Salt, Fresh Garlic, Fresh Parsley, Fresh Sage,
Fresh Chives, Fresh Basil
Oatmeal (About two - 1/2-Cup Servings)
Herbal Tea or Coffee Substitute
Nonfat Yogurt (Plain or Flavored)
Nonfat, Fruit Juice-Sweetened Granola
Puffed Brown Rice or Millet
Vegebase Powder
Orange Juice
Low-Fat Milk
Ice Cubes
Sunflower Seeds
Unroasted Pine Nuts
Raisins or Dried Currants
Extra-Virgin Olive Oil or Almond Oil, Canola Oil
TVP (Textured Vegetable Protein)
Slivered Almonds
Eggless, Low-Fat-Tofu-Based Mayonnaise
Brown Rice, Millet, Bulgur (Cracked Wheat)
Tempeh
Raw Sesame Seeds
Low Sodium Soy Sauce
Apple Cider Vinegar
Distilled Water
Whole Wheat Pasta
Filberts (or Other Nuts)

Soy Grits or Granules
Kelp
Soy Flour or Other Whole Grain Flour
Whole Wheat Pastry Flour
Whole Wheat Breadcrumbs
Crushed Tomatoes
Hot Pepper
Tomato Paste
Honey
Medium Tofu and Firm Tofu
Frozen Juice Concentrate
Alcohol-Free Vanilla Extract
Frozen Raspberries (10-Oz. Package)
Organically Grown Lemon Rind

# WEEK #2
# LIGHTEN UP WITH
# GENTLE JUICE CLEANSING

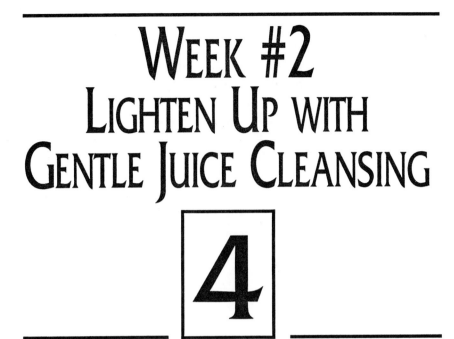

The second week of the 30-Day Body Purification Program is a consolidation of the information you used and loosely practiced during week 1. Now that you have had a chance to try out new foods and explore the purification process, this week will give you the opportunity to create more structure and afford you the opportunity to increase the elimination of accumulated waste products from your body.

During the next six days, you will be giving your body a rest from past dietetic mistakes and giving nature an opportunity to exert her wondrous ability to rebuild the body through a structured menu. On the final day of week 2, you will be using fruit and seed shakes in preparation for week 3 which consists primarily of juice fasting.

Many people find that physical afflictions that are aggravated by stressful situations are greatly eased or even eliminated after undergoing a program of juicing or juice fasting. Look over the following list for any health problems you or someone you love may have experienced. All of conditions have been associated with or are aggravated by high levels of stress. Juicing or juice fasting may be just what the doctor should be ordering for you to help clear away the extra toxins that your stressed-out body may be building up.

Human beings are complex organisms. We respond to stimuli emotionally, chemically and structurally, and spiritually. As a result excessive stress can effect us on many levels. Some of the health problems that can be reduced or eliminated with a reduction of stress include:

## TWENTY HEALTH PROBLEMS ASSOCIATED WITH ABNORMAL STRESS

1. Aches and pains
2. Diarrhea
3. Certain types of arthritis
4. Sexual problems
5. Alcoholism
6. Mood swings
7. Asthma
8. Lethargy
9. Backache
10. Reduced immunological function
11. Canker sores
12. Insomnia
13. Headaches
14. Dermatitis and other skin disorders
15. Hypertension
16. Colitis
17. Ulcers and other gastrointestinal disorders
18. Cardiovascular disease
19. Diabetes
20. Bruxism (jaw grinding)

## STRESS AND YOUR NERVOUS SYSTEM

Of all your body's systems, the nervous system is the most fragile. Its delicate balance is easily affected by a buildup of body toxins. Poor diet, as well as poor water, air, and noise quality or a combination of these factors, can create destructive stress. As a result of an imbalance of emotional, physical, or chemical factors, and the buildup of body toxins resulting from them, you may suffer from insomnia, nervous tension, and a host of other disorders.

Although we may tend to automatically consider stress and tension as harmful, they are essential parts of our everyday lives and are actually necessary for a balanced, productive existence. Consider, for example, the fact that both sex and laughter create a certain amount of stress and then provide a release of stress.

Stress may even help fight cancer. Research studies show that the body reacts to stress by increasing "its production of natural opiates called beta-endorphines, which appear to stimulate antitumor lymphocytes. These cells aid the body in fighting cancer by their role in activating the body's immune system" (Richard D. Lyons, "Stress Addiction: 'Life in the Fast Lane' May Have Its Benefits," *The New York Times*, July 26, 1983, Section C, p. 9.). So you see that stress can be beneficial, but only in moderate quantities.

Stress in immoderate quantities, on the other hand, overloads the body's resources and can be very harmful. If the body cannot handle the stress overload, it may reach with a "pathological" tension. When this tension increases, your breathing may become very shallow. Shallow breathing has a pronounced effect on the blood circulation throughout the body and reduces the amount of oxygen that reaches the brain. In addition to shallow breathing, your muscles will tighten up, especially around your pelvis, neck, and shoulders.

The following list will help you clarify how stressful your life is. If you have *high stress patterns* then this is an opportunity to make small changes that will lead you to a stress-free life.

## TESTING YOURSELF FOR STRESS

1. A healthy breathing pattern should be deep and regular. Do you have a healthy breathing pattern, or are your breaths shallow and erratic?
2. Do you stop during the day to become aware of the way you are breathing?
3. Comfortable clothing that does not bind by waist, chest, or

throat promotes healthy breathing. What type of clothing do you wear?

4. It is important to sit in a relaxed, upright position with your spine relatively straight and your legs uncrossed. Do you sit this way or do you slouch and cross your legs?

5. When you are not feeling well, you should pay special attention to relaxing and breathing deeply. Do you do this, or are you rushing to get things done in spite of how you feel.

6. Daily meditation and visualization exercises are important. Do you have enough time to meditate 15 or 20 minutes each day.

7. Exercise is essential to good health. Do you take 20 minutes daily to exercise?

8. Do you enjoy your job? if not do you explore ways to make it more emotionally satisfying?

9. Relaxation is very important. Do you make time every day to relax? Can you relax without feeling guilty about not working or not taking care of something important?

10. It's important to take a vacation now and then. Do you take vacations? Do you think about work while on vacation?

11. It's important to relax at meals and chew your food slowly. Do eat your meals in this way or do you eat in a hurry?

12. Are you at peace with yourself?

13. Caring and loving relationships are essential for physical and emotional health. Are your personal relationships satisfying?

14. Having good friends is one way of reducing stress. You can let off steam with them and get good advice. Do you listen to the opinions of others, or do you think you have all the answers?

15. The need to smoke or pick your nails are indications that you are high stress. What habits do you have that are related to stress.

16. Clear communication is a simple way to reduce stress. Do speak very quickly and rush through the ends of your sentences, or do you take the time to say what you need to slowly and articulately?

17. Learning to manage time is an important skill. Do you believe time management means "doing more things in less time"? Usually try to do two things at once?
18. Do you enjoy what you do to manage your stress.

### *Factors Contributing To Your Wellness*

1. Lifestyle
2. Personality Typology
3. Nutrition
4. Exercise
5. Stress Management
6. Relaxation
7. Reduction and Elimination of High-Risk Behavior
   A. Smoking
   B. Alcohol Consumption
   C. Overconsumption of Drugs
   D. Caffeine
8. Environmental Factors
   A Clean Air
   B. Clean Water
9. Adequate Sleep
10. Proper Weight
11. Satisfying And Challenging Work
12. Satisfying Interpersonal Relationships
13. Spiritual Attunement
14. Personal And Professional Growth
15. Love And Affection
16. Positive Thinking
17. Attitude And Belief System
18. Goals And Aspirations

HOW MEDITATION, PRAYER, AND EXERCISE WILL IMPROVE YOUR LIFE

*Marvin M. was an overweight asthmatic and mature-onset diabetic with a high-stress job. He was fearful that he might lose his eyesight due to his diabetes. Though he was not yet required to take insulin to control his blood sugar, this is what the future seemed to hold. Weak of will and virtually devoid of discipline, Marvin, due to the influence of his loving wife Carol, began to ask for the help of the divine power by praying every morning and evening. "Please, Lord," he said, "if it be your will, allow me the will power to heal and be healthy again." In addition to his praying, Marvin would sit quietly and practice visualization and meditation exercises. Slowly he would inhale and exhale, watching his breath as he did so. After 10 minutes or so he would go out for brisk 30-minute walk with Carol. Marvin's praying and mediation seemed to bring miracles. He enjoyed his daily walks, but in addition to this, he felt greater love and joy in his life and found it easier to avoid the junky, refined foods that he previously craved. Instead he began the 30-Day Purification Program. Within three weeks, Marvin's blood sugar level dropped and his breathing became much easier. He has not had an asthma attack since.*

## EASY WAYS TO AVOID EXCESS SUGAR

Approximately 75 percent of the sugar and other sweeteners in the typical American diet come from processed foods. It is important for body purification that you reduce your sugar consumption. The best way to do this is to learn where it's all coming from so you can know what to avoid or eliminate.

Confectionery products, any cereal and bakery products that are not whole grain, and most soft drinks contain refined sugar. The areas in which to cut back are quite obvious. It is essential that you read labels carefully. Avoid foods in which sugar, corn syrup, and so on are printed at the top of the ingredients list, or those that list several different sweeteners in a single product. Begin to question the presence of sugar in nearly everything you eat. The actual amount used in any one food may be small. But the point is, these small amounts do add up to far more than you should have.

## THREE BENEFITS OF REDUCING YOUR SUGAR INTAKE

1. Fewer "empty calories" in your diet
2. Less tooth decay
3. Less stress to your liver, adrenal glands, and pancreas

## HOW BODY PURIFICATION HELPED RICHARD S. MANAGE HIS DIABETES

*Richard S. was 45. He held a high stress job, smoked ciga-rettes, had a few beers every evening and was at least thirty pounds overweight. For the last year he had been experiencing excessive thirst, frequent urination and sexual impotence.*

*With coaxing from his wife he went to see a holistic physician. After performing blood and urine analysis, the doctor informed Richard that he had what is called Type 2 Diabetes. Formerly known as mature or adult onset diabetes, this condition resulted from the body's inability to manufacture or utilize insulin prop-erly. The good news was that if Richard S. could reduce his stress and develop a healthier lifestyle, the diabetes could be controlled.*

*The program he was given included the following suggestions:*

- *Prepare meals with more nonstarchy vegetables like sun-chokes, green leafy vegetables, sea vegetables, celery peppers and cabbage. Do not rely exclusively on starchy foods like beans, corn, and peas.*
- *Replace the beer with an alcohol free malt beverage.*
- *Join a "quit smoking" program while using the hydrothera-py program of cleansing baths to remove nicotine from the system.*
- *Increase intake of EFAS (essential fatty acids)by taking flax seed oil and forage oil supplementation. These EFAS can help the body normalize many biochemical abnormalities associated with diabetes.*
- *Eat high fiber foods especially whole grains. They reduce the insulin requirements for some diabetics.*
- *Practice aerobic exercise at least three times per week for twenty minutes a session.*

*Richard S. took his physician's advice. By his next birthday his weight had come down and his condition was under control. Thanks to his new body purifying lifestyle.*

## GETTING OFF THAT DIETING SEE-SAW WITH FRUITS AND JUICES

*Ronnie S. had struggled to lose weight by going from diet to diet. She would lose the weight, but then put it all back on again. She was finally able to lose inches from her waistline by using my three step program. On this easy 3 step program, Ronnie S. found that she had a natural control for her appetite while feeding her sweet tooth in a natural and healthy way. Each morning she would have a 16-oz. glass of carrot and beet juice. Throughout the day she would alternate fresh fruit salads with vegetables juices. Ronnie S. lost her excess weight and felt youthful, healthy, and fulfilled.*

## LEWIS HARRISON'S INTERNAL ORGAN PURIFICATION TEA

Combine:
1 Tablespoon Each of
    Mullein
      Spearmint
3/4 Tablespoon Each of
    Rose hips
      Orange peel
A Pinch of
    Golden seal

If you have access to a mail-order catalog for herbal teas or there is an herb store in your area, other herbs can be added to Purification Tea. These can include coltsfoot (an expectorant for lungs), fenugreek seeds (a demulcent for sore throat), papaya leaves (for digestive problems), blackberry root (diarrhea), buckthorn bark (for constipation), lemon grass (for taste), and red raspberry leaves (a tonic for pregnancy).

Mix equal amounts of spearmint and mullein. Since rose hips and orange peel are very intense to the taste, smaller amounts of these are used. Golden seal can be unpleasant tasting, but it is key to the formula. Use only a pinch. The effectiveness of this tea depends upon the amount of plant material used in relation to the amount of water used. A strong mixture will be brown in color; a weaker one will be yellow. One tablespoon of the herbs to one cup of distilled water makes a good average strength.

If you are making a large pot of Purification Tea, you can put the roots (golden seal) and dried fruit (rose hips) in the water as the temperature of the water increases to the boiling point. Add the leaves and orange peel as the water is about to boil. The essential oils in the herbs will burn out if they are boiled, so it is important to control the heat by turning it off. The mixture should steep for a couple of minutes. After you have consumed the pot of herbal tea, the herbs can be reused for a second pot, and a third, depending upon the strength of the mixture.

An alternative method of brewing is to place a few tablespoons of the Purification Tea herbal mixture into a strainer and pour boiling water over it and let it steep for a couple of minutes in the cup. This can be done several times before the mixture loses its potency. These are general guidelines, and any combination of any amount of the herbs can be blended together according to what is available and individual taste preferences. The important thing is that you use these herbs consistently during the rest of the 30-Day Program.

### HEALING A TOXIC LIVER AND BALANCING BLOOD SUGAR LEVELS WITH LEWIS'S TEA

*Lily E., now a healthy 75-year-old, came dangerously close in 1988 to being hospitalized. She was a plagued with low blood sugar and an inability to digest oil-rich foods. It was just two years ago that Lily began taking her health seriously. Until then, her health habits were very poor. She loved to eat fast foods, lots of sugar, and refined highly processed foods like white bread and white rice. One day she got dizzy and fainted on the New York City subway. When she came to, she went home. Only when his family prodded her did Lily finally visit a holistic physician, who immediately diagnosed the condition as a poor lifestyle, aggravating an already existing medical problem. Lily immediately began using the 30-Day Purification Program and drinking Lewis's tea daily. This program helped to heal her toxic liver and reduce her blood sugar problems.*

## THE POWERFUL HEALING OF JUICES AND TEAS

Freshly pressed juices having been used in just the last hundred years or so are among the more recently discovered natural healing tools. Juices are a great source of easily absorbed nutrients and plant essences and have a powerful effect on the body's recuperative powers. One of the most important aspects of fresh juice therapy is the amount of enzymes that they make available to the system. Plant food enzymes are the key to life and are extremely valuable on all levels of the healing and rehabilitation process. According to N. Walker, a pioneer in the use of juice therapy in the United States, "The juices extracted from fresh raw vegetables and fruits are the means by which we can furnish all the cells and tissues of the body with the elements and the nutritional enzymes which they need, in the manner in which they can be most readily digested and assimilated" (*Raw Vegetable Juices*, p. 14, by N. Walker, Pyramid Books). Digestive function, assimilation, and elimination are all assisted by the presence of enzymes. Enzymes help perform many biological processes without energy and without becoming involved in the processes themselves. These enzymes serve as catalysts that help the body go on with its healing.

### Four Tips to Obtain the Greatest Healing Value from Juices

1. Use only freshly extracted juices as described in the section of the appendix called "Your Home Guide to Juicing." Canned and bottled juices are of limited or no value in a juice therapy program.
2. Drink juice immediately after it is extracted. Do not refrigerate or store it for later use.
3. Use fruits and vegetables that are fresh. Green vegetables should have a full color. Avoid iceberg lettuce, blanched celery, etcetera
4. Drink about a pint of juice daily if you are in a generally healthy state. If you are ill or on a purification program, it may be appropriate, depending on the particular formula used to take 16-oz. portions of juice at least two to four times daily. Certain juices seem to have their greatest effect when combined with other juices. Among these are the juice of asparagus, beets and beet greens, dandelion, garlic, horseradish root, lemon, parsley, radish, spinach, and turnips.

### THE VITAMIN AND MINERAL BLOOD-BUILDING BENEFITS OF FRESH EXTRACTED JUICES

Freshly pressed juices are rich in proteins, carbohydrates, enzymes, chlorophyll, aromatic oils, and other important healing and purifying components. They are also a great source of easily absorbed nutrients and plant essences and have a powerful effect on the bodies recuperative powers. The following list will offer many of the purifying and healing elements to be found in fresh fruits and vegetables. Just juice them and drink their magic healing powers.

*Apples:* Pectin, potassium, phosphorus, cellulose. Lowers blood pressure. Eliminates constipation.

*Asparagus:* An effective diuretic, this juice is very healing to the kidneys. It is especially valuable for breaking up oxalic acids accumulations throughout the body.

*Beets:* Potassium. Used by many healers as a blood building tool.

*Beet greens:* Vitamin A, potassium, calcium, iron.

*Blueberry:* Astringent, antiseptic, blood purifier.

*Brussel sprouts:* A regenerator for pancreatic function and digestion.

*Cabbage:* Sulphur, chlorine, iodine. A great cleanser for the mucous membranes of the intestines and stomach.

*Carrots:* Beta-carotene, potassium, sodium, calcium, magnesium, iron. The highest source among juices for beta-carotene, a powerful aid to the maintenance of the bones and teeth. Of special value for disorders of the liver and intestines.

*Celery:* Potassium, sodium, calcium, phosphorus, magnesium.

*Cucumber:* Chlorine, sulphur, silicon. Probably the most powerful diuretic among the juices.

*Dandelion:* Potassium, calcium, sodium, magnesium, iron. Used to counteract hyperacidity in the system.

*Fennel (Finocchio):* A powerful blood builder.

*Garlic:* Extremely rich in mustard oils. A powerful cleanser of mucous from the sinus cavities and bronchial tubes. Garlic is best taken mixed with other milder juices.

*Grapefruit:* Vitamin C, potassium.

*Kale:* Used the same as cabbage juice.

*Leek:* Used the same as garlic or onion juice. Leek juice is much milder.

*Lemon:* Vitamin C, bioflavinoids. Powerful cleanser of mucous.

*Onion:* Used the same as garlic juice. Onion juice is much milder.

*Parsnip (Cultivated, Not Wild):* Chlorine, potassium, phosphorus, silicon, sulphur.

*Papaya:* Though delicious when ripe, the juice of the unripe papaya is high in papain, a protein digesting enzyme. According to N.W. Walker, the juice of unripe papaya also contains fibrin, an element that is valuable in the coagulation or clotting of the blood.

*Parsley:* Vitamin C, Vitamin A, calcium magnesium, phosphorus, potassium. Especially of value for the adrenal and thyroid glands.

*Potato:* Chlorine, phosphorus, potassium, sulphur. Eliminates muscle cramps.

*Radish:* Potassium, sodium, iron, magnesium. Blood builder.

*Sorrel:* Iron, magnesium, phosphorus, sulphur, silicon. Builds nails and healthy hair.

*Tomato:* Sodium, calcium, potassium, magnesium. Builds strong bones and healthy gums.

*Turnip:* Turnip leaves may have highest level of calcium of all juicing vegetables. Builds strong bones.

## JUICING IS EVEN MORE PURIFYING THAN FASTING

The rich and famous love to go to health spas, and today, almost all the European health spas and clinics use juice-fasting. Most of the leading authorities on health and nutrition agree that fasting on fresh, raw fruit and vegetable juices, with the addition of vegetable broth and herb teas, will result in a faster recovery from disease and more effective cleansing of toxic wastes than will a water fast. Now you can bring the spa into your home by juicing daily.

Raw juices are rich in vitamins, organic minerals, trace elements, and enzymes. These vital elements are easily assimilated without straining the digestive system, helping to accelerate the regeneration of the cells and overall recovery of the body.

Dr. Ragnar Berg, a world-famous authority on nutrition and biochemistry, said:

> During fasting the body burns up and excretes huge amounts of accumulated wastes. We can help this cleansing process by drinking alkaline juices instead of water while fasting. I have supervised many fasts and made extensive examinations and tests of fasting patients, and I am convinced that drinking alkaline-forming fruit and vegetable juices, instead of water, during the fasting is functionally much better. Elimination of uric acid and other inorganic acids will be accelerated. And the sugars in juices will strengthen the heart. Juice fasting is, therefore, the best form of fasting.

If you use the juice purification program, you will discover how much more energy and vitality you can have. Juice purification is an easy and efficient way to improve your skin tone and give you a sense of lightness on your feet. Juicing is a great way to lose weight, while cleansing your bloodstream and vital organs.

## SEVEN DAYS OF PURIFICATION WITH ENZYME-RICH JUICES

Here is my favorite juice program. Try it for a day or two and if you like it then continue for up to seven days. If you find it too difficult to apply then repeat the menu from week 2.

Upon Rising
*One 8-oz. glass of freshly squeezed citrus juice (orange or grapefruit) or 1/2 lemon, squeezed into a glass of distilled water. This is rich in vitamin C, which helps to strengthen your blood vessels.*

Midmorning
*One cup of Purification Tea with a small amount of honey if desired.*

This will flush out toxins from your internal organs.

Noontime
*One large glass of freshly extracted Basic Cleansing Juice consisting of carrot-celery-parsley.*

This is rich in minerals and beta-carotene. These strengthen the immune system.

Evening
*A bowl of warm potassium broth or a glass of fresh vegetable juice. This helps replenish the body's minerals.*

Before Retiring
*A cup of Purification Tea with a small amount of honey, if desired.*

If you wish, Purification Tea can be alternated with other milder teas, such as peppermint, chamomile, and rose hips. All three of these herbs have healing properties. Chamomile is a relaxant and is superb for the digestive system. It makes a good nighttime tea. Rose hips has a high content of Vitamin C, which is helpful in detoxifying during fasting. Peppermint is an excellent overall restorative herb.

Carrot-celery-parsley is an excellent combination. The ideal combination is 5 parts carrot, 2 parts celery, and 1/2 part parsley. (Parsley should be taken in small quantities due to its high iron content.) Carrot-apple is another popular combination. Combine in any part distribution you desire. These formulas help flush out the kidneys.

If you want to expand beyond just juicing, try a vegetable broth made by gathering various vegetables (potatoes, carrots, broccoli, string beans, cauliflower, celery, turnips, cabbage, onions, sea vegetables, etcetera), cooking them in distilled water in a large pot for about 30 minutes (low flame), and straining the broth. This broth is cleansing and health building at the same time.

When thirsty, drink distilled water with fresh lemon juice added to taste. Your total juice and broth intake for the day should be between one and one and one-half quarts.

Mild exercise during the day will highly benefit you during your juice fast. Walking, stretching, or yoga if you are used to it, are excellent forms of exercise.

HOW A DRUMMER LIGHTENED UP HIS "LEAD BELLY'
(WITH JUICING)

*Norman B. is interested in getting rid of his "spare tire." A compulsive overeater he needed the discipline of a "natural foods" program without the food. Juicing was the answer. Norman B. made the commitment by going on a four-week juicing program.*

*He prepared by eating nothing but fresh fruits and vegetables for a week. He felt more motivated as he saw how he looked thinner as the days went by. At the beginning of the week he began drinking 20 oz. of fresh juice three times a day. At the end of the four-week schedule, he felt great and had lost the excess weight he had been carrying in his abdomen.*

**WEEK 2 DAILY MENU PLANS, EXERCISES, AND MEDITATIONS**
*Menu Plan*

**Day 8**

Breakfast                    *16 oz. Juice Formula #3\**
                             *1 cup fresh fruit salad — oranges, grapefruit,*
                             *tangerine*

*Herbal tea or coffee substitute*

Lunch

*1 bowl of Spicy Garden Vegetable Soup\**
*1 mixed vegetable salad consisting of*
*1 cup chopped cucumber*
*1 medium tomato, sliced*
*2 cups romaine lettuce*
*Red Garlic Dressing\**
*Herbal tea or coffee substitute*

Dinner

*1 bowl of miso soup*
*1/2 cup brown rice with Tomato Sauce\**
*1/2 cup lentils*
*1 cup of a steamed, pleasant-tasting sea vegetable (arame, wakamae, kombu, hijiki, nori)*
*1/2 cup steamed carrots*
*1 cup steamed cauliflower*

## Arm Circles

This exercise helps to relieve tension in your shoulders and neck, strengthening shoulders and arms.

1. Stand with your feet at shoulder width, your arms horizontal, parallel with the floor, and your palms facing sky.

2. Move your arms in small circles, from back to front.

3. Increase the size of the circle as much as possible.

4. Repeat ten circles.

5. Decrease size the circles until your arms become parallel with floor in the tenth circle (starting point).

6. Reverse direction and repeat step 2-5

Do not drop arms between steps 4 and 5. Remember to keep taking long full breaths into your abdomen.

---

\*Recipes for starred beverages, main dishes, soups, and sauces may be found in Appendix IV, "Herbs and Spices," Appendix V, "Your Home Guide to Juicing," and Appendix VII," "Purification Recipes"

*Menu Plan*

**Day 9**

Breakfast
> *Berry Heaven Blended Cocktail\**
> *1 cup fresh fruit salad — oranges, grapefruit, tangerines*
> *Herbal tea or coffee substitute*

Lunch
> *1 bowl of Spicy Garden Vegetable Soup\**
> *1 mixed vegetable salad consisting of*
> > *1 cup grated carrots*
> > *1 medium tomato, sliced*
> > *2 cups romaine lettuce*
> > *Tahini Dressing\**
> *Herbal tea or coffee substitute*

Dinner
> *1 bowl of miso soup*
> *1/2 cup millet with Soy-Tomato Sauce\**
> *1/2 cup chick peas*
> *1 cup of a steamed, pleasant-tasting sea vegetable (arame, wakamae, kombu, hijiki, nori)*
> *1 cup steamed cauliflower*

## Contraction-Relaxation (The Arms)

This exercise is great for increasing your energy levels and reducing fatigue.

1. Lie down on your back.
2. Focus your attention to your right hand.
3. Rotate your thumb and fingers; open and close your palm. Stretch fingers and palm. (The center of palm will rise slightly.) Hold for one breath.
4. Make a fist and rotate from your wrist; create pressure for one breath.
5. Straighten your arm off floor 2 inches.
6. Tense your fist, forearm, and upper arm as tight as you can for one breath and relax it.
7. Roll the arm back and forth.
8. Repeat steps 2-7 with left hand and arm.

*Menu Plan*

**Day 10**

Breakfast
> *16 oz. Juice Formula #3\**
> *1 cup fresh fruit salad — Oranges, grape fruit, tangerines*
> *Herbal tea or coffee substitute*

Lunch
> *1 bowl of Spicy Garden Vegetable Soup*
> *1 mixed vegetable salad consisting of*
> > *1 cup chopped cucumber*
> > *1 medium tomato, sliced*
> > *1 cups romaine lettuce*
> > *1/2 cup grated carrots*
> > *1 cup alfalfa sprouts*
> > *Sweet Dill Dressing\**
> *Herbal tea or coffee substitute*

Dinner
> *1 bowl of miso soup*
> *Tofu Vegetable Casserole\**
> *1 cup of a steamed, pleasant-tasting sea vegetable (arame, wakamae, kombu, hijiki, nori) with Black Bean Sauce\**
> *1/2 cup steamed carrots*
> *1 ear of corn on the cob*

## Contraction/Relaxation (The Rectum and Upper Body)

This is great exercise for increasing your energy levels and reducing fatigue.

1. Lie down on your back.
2. Focus your attention on your rectum.
3. Contract the muscles in your rectum. If done correctly, your buttocks will rise from the ground.
4. Tighten for one breath. Exhale and relax.
5. Inhale long and deep into your abdomen.
6. Holding your breath for three counts, push out your abdomen. Exhale rapidly through mouth.

7. After 10 seconds of normal breathing, expand your chest. Push out from inside, holding the breath for three counts; exhale rapidly.

*Menu Plan*

**Day 11**

Breakfast
*High-Protein Fruit Smoothie\**
*1 cup fresh pineapple*
*Herbal tea or coffee substitute*

Lunch
*1 bowl of vegetable bouillon*
*(available from health food store)*
*1 mixed vegetable salad consisting of*
*1 cup chopped cucumber*
*1 medium tomato, sliced*
*1 cups romaine lettuce*
*1/2 cup grated carrots*
*1 cup alfalfa sprouts*
*Green Garlic Dressing\**
*Herbal tea or coffee substitute*

Dinner
*1 bowl of E-Z ABC Soup\**
*1/2 cup kasha*
*1/2 cup white beans*
*1 cup of a steamed, pleasant-tasting*
*sea vegetable*
*(arame, wakamae, kombu, hijiki, nori)*
*1/2 cup baked butternut squash*
*1 cup steamed broccoli*

## Wrist Circles

This exercise is great for stimulating and strengthening your entire arm, including wrist, forearms, and shoulders. It is also valuable for stretching your thighs and ankles.

1. Sit in on the back of your legs and heels, with the top of your feet (instep) flat on the floor.
2. Raise your arms to a horizontal position with your elbows slightly bent, and with your palms facing each other.

3. Circle your hands, palms out, from wrist five times toward the inside-right hand moving counterclockwise, left hand clockwise.

4. Inhale during step 3.

5. Circle hands from wrist five times toward the outside-right hand moving clockwise, left hand counterclockwise. Exhale five times.

Repeat steps 2-5 four times. Add two rounds each week until you are doing ten. Feel the pressure on your wrist. Breathe into your abdomen.

*Menu Plan*

**Day 12**

Breakfast

*16 oz. Juice Formula #3*
*1 cup fresh fruit salad — Apples, pears,*
   *plums*
*Herbal tea or coffee substitute*

Lunch

*1 bowl of miso soup with 1/2 cup mung*
   *bean sprouts*
*1 mixed vegetable salad consisting of:*
   *1 cup grated zucchini squash*
   *1 medium tomato, sliced*
   *2 cups romaine lettuce*
   *1/2 cup grated carrots*
   *1 cup alfalfa sprouts*
   *Ginger Peanut Dressing**
*Herbal tea or coffee substitute*

Dinner

*1 bowl of miso soup*
*1/2 cup brown rice*
*1/2 cup textured vegetable protein*
*1 cup of a steamed, pleasant-tasting*
   *sea vegetable (arame, wakamae, kombu,*
   *hijiki, nori) with Chinese Sweet Mustard*
   *Sauce**
*1/2 cup steamed pumpkin*
*1 cup steamed cauliflower*

## Visualization Technique: A Basic Approach to Stress Reduction and Relaxation

Step 1. Find a quiet place where you will not be disturbed.

Step 2. Sit in a straight-backed chair, with both feet flat on the floor and your hands facing palms up and resting on your knees.

Step 3. Close your eyes and inhale and exhale long and slowly.

Step 4. As you exhale, visualize that you are actually exhaling out the stress and tension from your body.

Step 5. Finish this visualization by taking a long deep breath, slowly exhaling and gradually opening your eyes. Remain quiet for a few minutes, becoming aware of your surroundings without getting up or moving around.

Step 6. Slowly begin to wiggle your toes and fingers.

Step 7. When you feel acclimated to the surrounding environment you can arise.

*Menu Plan*

### Day 13

Breakfast              *16 oz. Juice Formula #3*
*1 cup tropical fresh fruit salad — banana, mango, papaya*
*Herbal tea or coffee substitute*

Lunch                  *1 bowl of Spicy Garden Vegetable Soup\**
*1 mixed cold sea vegetable salad consisting of 1/2 cup each of*
*Kombu*
*Arame*
*Wakame*
*Nori*
*Macrobiotic Twig Tea\* or other herbal teas substitute*

Dinner                 *1 bowl of miso soup with 1/2 cup soba (buckwheat) noodles*
*1/2 cup black beans*

> 1 cup of a steamed, pleasant-tasting
>   sea vegetable (arame, wakamae, kombu,
>   hijiki, nori)
> 1/2 cup steamed carrots
> 1 cup steamed cauliflower

## Yoga Shoulder Release

This yoga exercise to loosen stiff shoulders and tight upper back muscles.

1. Stand with your feet 6 inches apart and your arms at your sides.
2. Wrap your your fingers around your thumbs, making a fist.
3. Straighten your arms imagining a stiff pole connecting shoulder to thumbs.
4. Inhale, raising your shoulders as high as possible.
5. Tighten your shoulders.
6. Exhale, dropping shoulders quickly, and relax.

Start with 20 breath/releases; add 2 per session until you reach 50.

*Menu Plan*

**Day 14**

Breakfast

> 16 oz. Juice Formula #3
> 1 cup fresh fruit salad — Oranges, grape
>   fruit, tangerines
> Herbal tea or coffee substitute

Lunch

> 1 bowl of Spicy Garden Vegetable Soup*
> A mixed dill and sprout salad consisting of:
>   1 cup chopped cucumber
>   1 medium tomato, sliced
>   1 cups sunflower sprouts
>   1/2 cup grated carrots
>   1 cup alfalfa sprouts
>   Sweet Dill Dressing
> Herbal tea or coffee substitute

Dinner

> 1 bowl of miso soup
> 1/2 cup brown rice

*1/2 cup lentils*
*1 cup of a steamed, pleasant tasting*
*sea vegetable (arame, wakamae, kombu,*
*hijiki, nori)*
*1/2 cup steamed carrots*
*1 cup steamed green peas*

## Chest Toner

This isometric (toning) exercise gives strength and shape to the pectoral muscles that support the breast. It also helps strengthen the upper arms.

1. Stand with your feet 6 inches apart, with your elbows bent, and hands clasped in front of your chest at shoulder level, as if to clap.
2. Press the heel of your palms together while creating palm-to-palm pressure.
3. Inhale while pressing. Hold for three counts. Exhale while releasing.

Start with 10 of these; add 10 a week until you reach 50. Remember to keep elbows up at shoulder level.

## SUGGESTED GROCERY LIST FOR WEEK 2

*Fresh Vegetables*: Onion, celery, green pepper, medium tomatoes, carrots, romaine lettuce, cucumbers, onions, cauliflower, alfalpha sprouts, fresh or frozen peas, zucchini, scallions, corn on the cob, white potatoes, butternut squash, mung bean sprouts, pumpkin, carrots, celery, cabbage
*Fresh Fruit*: Oranges, grapefruits, tangerines, apples, pears, pineapple, plums, banana, mango, papaya, blueberries (fresh or unsweetened frozen), strawberries (fresh or unsweetened frozen), lemon
*Spices (dried)*: ginger powder, garlic powder, cayenne pepper powder, onion powder, dry mustard, dried basil, dried parsley or soup herbs, bay leaf, white or black pepper corns, sea salt (optional), dried rosemary, sea salt (optional)
Whole natural sunflower seeds

Almond oil or extra-virgin olive oil

Vegebase or vegetable powder

Prepared miso soup or, if making miso soup from scratch, miso paste and distilled water.

Brown rice(short-grain); otherwise whatever is available

Extra virgin olive oil, sesame oil, and canola oil

*Fresh herbs*: garlic, fresh oregano, fresh basil, fresh parsley, fresh dill, fresh ginger

Crushed tomatoes

Six Servings Of Sea Vegetable(s):Arame, wakamae, kombu, hijiki, nori—one or as many as desired

Low-fat milk

Ice cubes (if some on hand)

Herbal tea or coffee substitute for everyday use

Macrobiotic twig tea (or other herbal tea)

Red wine vinegar

Apple cider vinegar

Distilled water

Tahini

Tamari

Millet

Kasha

Whole grain alphabet pasta

Soba (buckwheat noodles)

Light soy sauce

Chick peas

Lentils

Black beans

Dijon mustard

Honey

Firm tofu and soft tofu

Rice wine or sherry

Cornstarch or arrowroot powder

Fresh hot chilies

Unsweetened frozen fruit

Pure vanilla extract
Ice cubes (if some available)
Soy mayonnaise
White beans
Natural peanut butter
Textured vegetable protein
Sunflower seeds

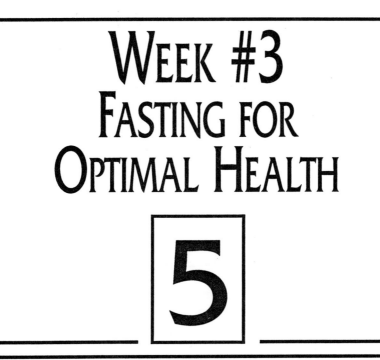

# WEEK #3
## FASTING FOR
## OPTIMAL HEALTH

Fasting has been used for thousands of years as a means of physical and spiritual cleansing and purification. Programs that limit food intake to teas, juices, or broths are called fasts.

For most of the last two centuries, spas in Switzerland, Germany and Austria were the fasting centers of the world. Reports of 30- and 40-day fasts on water and nothing else were not uncommon.

In the last few years, this has begun to change. Fasting has become very popular in the United States. Many body purification specialists have been adding broths and juices to fasting regimes. This shift is largely due to an increase in the use of pesticides, insecticides, fungicides, and other potentially toxic chemicals by farmers, as well as the increase in air and water pollution. These chemical agents tend to accumulate in the body, and water fasting may result in their being released into the bloodstream too rapidly. Many health professionals have told me that their clients have been experiencing symptoms during water fasts that they have not seen in past years such as nausea and diarrhea. The only explanation that they have for this is the possibility of high levels of toxic chemicals in the bloodstream. Among the symptoms reported on these water fasts are dizziness, blurry vision, leg pains, and headaches. *For this reason, it is best to use modified fasts with herbal teas, vegetable broths, juices, and other healing liquids.*

Traditionally, fasting is done in conjunction with steam baths, special showers, breathing exercises, and the drinking of herbal teas and freshly pressed juices. One way of increasing the effectiveness of a fast, and the cleansing process it creates is to use a broad spectrum of fiber sources, antioxidants, and herbal teas for cleansing and flushing out internal organs.

## TWELVE IMPORTANT BENEFITS OF FASTING

Fasting has been used as a healing and purifying technique since the beginning of recorded time. There are thousands of recognized benefits to fasting. Twelve of the most important are listed below.

1. Cleanses the body of metabolic wastes and other poisonous and toxic substances.
2. Accelerates elimination or detoxification process.
3. Empties the digestive tract and disposes of putrefactive bacteria.
4. Restores youthful conditioning of the cells and tissues.
5. Rejuvenates the entire body.
6. Elevates energy levels.
7. Promotes harmonious functioning of all body parts.
8. Adds to peace of mind.
9. Promotes efficient digestion and assimilation.
10. Heightens sense perception.
11. Strengthens mental power.
12. Normalizes high blood pressure.

How Intelligent Fasting Helped a Computer Operator Lose 20 Pounds in 30 Days

*Gladys P. was interested in taking off the excess weight she had gained during the year she had managed a restaurant on South Beach in Miami. She needed the self-discipline of a regularly scheduled program and wanted to cleanse her system as well. Fasting seemed like the perfect choice. She set herself a goal of intense cleansing over a four-week period. By a combination of water, vegetable broths, and light consistent walking, she was able to achieve her goal. At the end of the fast, she readjusted her body by going on the 30-Day Purification Program.*

## WHAT SCIENTISTS SAY ABOUT FASTING

The basic theory behind fasting is that through these techniques, there is an increase in the elimination of waste matter, as well as the passing of metabolic wastes through the skin, the lungs, the kidneys, the bowels, and the other avenues of elimination. Though there is general interest on the subject of fasting, there has been little interest in the medical community to study the benefits of fasting in controlled studies. Most of what is known about fasting is based on what is said by those who have fasted and by anecdotal reports of nutritionists who use this approach. In the last two decades, some studies have been conducted that indicate that fasting may have therapeutic benefits in treating various disorders, including

Rheumatoid arthritis

Obesity—a juice and herbal tea fast was used here

Headaches due to allergies

## BEFORE YOU DECIDE TO FAST: WHO SHOULD NOT FAST

You should not fast if you have any of the following conditions. Check with your doctor or natural health practitioner if you are unsure of your condition.

A tendency or predisposition to thrombosis and blood diseases

Heart disease

Low blood pressure

Anorexia

Bulimia

Tumors

Bleeding ulcers

Certain types of cancer

Juvenile diabetes

Gout

Liver disease

Kidney disease

Recent myocardial infarction

Pregnancy

Any condition requiring long-term medication

A new mother, unless she has been examined by a competent health professional and told that her uterus is back in its prepregnancy state

Children

Nursing women

## PREPARING YOUR BODY FOR A FAST

Some people will fast one day per week as a matter of habit. According to some authorities on fasting, the body will always tell you when it should be rested and allowed to detoxify. One such sign is the "coated tongue." A yellow, green, or thick off-white coating on your tongue is considered to be a sign of autointoxication. Lab tests have shown that these coatings can serve as a medium for mold, yeast, and bacteria, indicating a low resistance to disease. As a person fasts, this coating may initially get worse and then slowly disappear.

In the early stages of a fast, an individual may experience acidosis of the blood, low blood sugar, depression, fatigue, or excess energy. Sometimes these reactions can be frightening. It is for this reason that you limit an unsupervised fast to no more than two or three days. Fasting must be done with care so that it never lasts long enough to cause nutritional deficiencies, loss of healthy tissue, or damage to the vital organs.

At least two quarts of liquid should be taken daily. This may be in the form of fresh vegetable juice, a combination of vegetable and fruit juices, potassium broth, water, or herbal teas. Potassium broths are highly alkaline liquids, often used during a fast to combat the acidosis (high acidity) of the blood as well as the acidosis of the body tissues that often occurs at the start of a purification program. Potassium broths are also very popular because they are nutrient rich and tasty! Boil potatoes, string beans, celery and zucchini in distilled water. When cooked, blend the entire mixture. This broth will help counteract the acidity if it occurs during a fast.

## STARTING A SIMPLE FAST

1. For three to four days prior to the fast, limit your foods to fresh fruits and vegetables, with about 8 oz. of plain yogurt or buttermilk.
2. When you are ready to begin the fast, start with freshly pressed vegetable juices. Concentrate on the green leafy vegetables, as well as beets. Use 1 quart a day, plus another 24 oz. of an herbal cleansing tea, such as red clover or ginger, and 16 oz. of an alkaline potassium broth.
3. After you have fasted for your desired time (up to three days), you can prepare to break the fast.

NOTE: *Supervised fasts have been known to be as long as five or six weeks without negative effects. However, this should never be attempted without skilled supervision.*

REMEMBER: *Fasting should be done conservatively and responsibly. When you fast, the goal is to cleanse the toxins and metabolic wastes through the various organs of elimination at an increased rate, as well as resting both body and mind.*

## HOW TO END YOUR FAST

Do not binge or overeat after a fast. Your digestive system is sensitive and rested. Excessive or improper meal planning soon after a fast may cause diarrhea or constipation.

1. First Day After the Fast:

   *Breaking a Water Fast:* Take 4 oz. of fresh orange or grapefruit and mix it with 4 oz. of distilled water. Sip this amount every three hours.
   *Breaking a Juice, Herbal, or Broth Fast:* Use some fruit but chew it very slowly. The best choices are watermelon or citrus.

2. Second Day: You may add a small vegetable salad, brown rice or baked potatoes.

3. Third Day: You may add a small vegetable salad, brown rice or baked potatoes.
4. Fourth Day: Eat small lactovegetarian meals.

Breaking a fast that is more than two days is as vital to the fast as the juices themselves. You can ruin a fast if you do not break it in the proper way. When breaking a fast:

1. Do not overeat to the point of feeling full.
2. Eat slowly and chew your food thoroughly.
3. Take several days to gradually return to the normal diet (allow more or fewer days, depending on the length of the program).

If you decide to go on a three-day fast, this same plan of action can be followed with great results. If you fast three or more days on this program, you may wish to include enemas in the morning to increase the detoxifying action. Firm daily scrubbing with a loofah sponge or something similar will increase circulation, thus increasing detoxification, and will encourage the skin to shed dead cells.

Do not fast more than seven to ten days without professional supervision. Extended juice fasts have been known to last over a period of months, but these were conducted under strict supervision in spas or health clinics specializing in fasting.

When breaking a seven-to-ten-day fast:

On the first day, eat only a piece of fruit for breakfast and a small vegetable salad for dinner. Continue to drink the same amount of juices.

On the second day, eat fruit such as prunes, figs, or raisins that have been soaked in distilled water to help your bowels move naturally. Have a small salad at dinner and increase your fruit intake to two pieces during the course of the day. Continue with the juices.

On the third day, increase your salad portion and add low-fat cottage cheese, buttermilk, kefir, or yogurt. You may also add a handful of freshly shelled, raw, unsalted nuts and seeds and half a cup of a cooked whole grain. As you add more solid foods, it is important that you continue to drink a couple of glasses of fresh juice as a part of your regular purification program.

On the fourth day, start to eat normally, but do not eat to the point of feeling uncomfortable. Normal in this case would mean the eating guidelines described in week 2.

### FASTING FOR RELIEF FROM ARTHRITIS PAIN

*Earl F. was a 75-year-old heavy-set sculptor with arthritis pain in his hands and elbows. Hardly able to practice his art any longer, he came to me begging for help. I placed him on juice for a week and then on a water fast. Wanting to avoid a drastic reaction, I allowed him to have some fresh fruit when the desire became too strong and then back on the fast he went. Over the two weeks of the fast, the swelling in his hands diminished and the redness and inflammation diminished as well. Self-massage techniques were taught to him to increase circulation to the formerly inflamed areas. His condition remained satisfactory so long as he stayed on a whole foods program.*

# FASTING AND JUICING

A regimen of fasting combined with juicing can work wonders for those seeking to regain a sense of well being, experience greater vigor and regain a more youthful appearance. It will help revitalize your body and increase your feeling of aliveness. Let this program work for you and learn what truly healthy can mean.

## Cleansing the Organs with Herbal Teas

Use mild teas such as peppermint, chamomile, and rose hips. All three of these herbs have healing properties. Chamomile is a relaxant and is superb for the digestive system. It makes a good nighttime tea. Rose hips has a high content of vitamin C, which is helpful in detoxifying during fasting. Peppermint is an excellent overall restorative herb.

Your total fluid intake daily (consisting of juice, distilled water and broth) should be between one and one and one-half quarts.

## REMEMBER TO EXERCISE

Mild exercise during the day will highly benefit you during your juice fast. Walking, or jogging, if you are used to it, are excellent forms of exercise.

<u>**WEEK 3 DAILY MENU PLANS, EXERCISES, AND MEDITATIONS**</u>

*Day 15*

Upon Rising

*If combining your fast with some food, eat only a piece of fruit for breakfast and a small vegetable salad for dinner. Continue to drink the same amount of juices. If fasting, take one 8-oz. glass of freshly squeezed citrus juice (orange or grapefruit) or 1/2 lemon squeezed into a glass of dis tilled water. This is rich in vitamin C, which helps to strengthen your blood vessels.*

Midmorning

*Drink one cup of Purification Tea with a small amount of honey if desired. This will flush out toxins from your internal organs.*

Noontime

*Take one large glass of freshly extracted Basic Cleansing Juice\* consisting of carrot-celery parsley. This is rich in minerals and beta-carotene. These strengthen the immune system.*

Evening

*Eat a bowl of warm potassium broth or a glass of fresh vegetable juice. This helps replenish the body's minerals.*

Before Retiring

*Drink a cup of Purification Tea with small amount of honey if desired.*

**Breath Integration**

This exercise helps to integrate muscles and breathing to normal.

1. Stand with your feet 6 inches apart.
2. Clasp your fingers together in front of you, and let your arms relax.

---

\* Recipes for starred beverages, main dishes, soups, and sauces may be found in Appendix IV, "Herbs and Spices," Appendix V, "Your Home Guide to Juicing," and Appendix VII, "Purification Recipes."

3. Inhale deeply while you bring your clasped hands straight over your head. (As the arms move up on the inhalation, imagine them floating on the breath.)
4. Let your forearms fall behind your head.
5. Place a little pressure on the heels of your hands, and start your exhalation as your arms return to where they began in front of you.

## *Menu Plan*

### *Day 16*

| | |
|---|---|
| Upon Rising | *16-oz. Juice Cocktail #1** |
| Midmorning | *1 bowl of miso soup* |
| Noontime | *1 bowl of E-Z ABC Soup** |
| Evening | *16-oz. Juice Cocktail #17** |
| Before Retiring | *1 cup Purification Tea with a small amount of honey if desired* |

## Stimulate Eye Circulation

This exercise stretches and promotes circulation for your eye muscles. You can also use this exercise to bring relief to tired eyes.

1. Sit in a comfortable position on the floor on a chair.
2. Move your eyes horizontally right to left, left to right.
3. Move your eyes horizontally and vertically up and down.
4. Move your eyes horizontally and diagonally upper right to lower left and back.
5. Move your eyes diagonally, upper left to lower right and back.
6. Move your eyes in a letter "U" motion, from upper right down and up to upper left and back.
7. Move your eyes in a rainbowlike direction, swinging up from the lower right and down to lower left and back.
8. Rub your palms together, generating heat and place your palms on your eyes for five seconds.

9. Lightly stroke your eyelids from side to side with your fin-
gertips (do this twice).

Repeat each eye movement three times, stretching to the extremes
but don't strain. Close your eyes for a moment between each exercise but stay still and don't move your head.

*Menu Plan*

**Day 17**

Upon Rising           *16-oz. Juice Cocktail #3\**

Midmorning         *1 cup Purification Tea with a small amount
of honey, if desired.*

Noontime            *1 bowl of Spicy Garden Vegetable Soup\**

Evening             *16-oz. Juice Cocktail #2*

Before
Retiring             *1 bowl of miso soup*

## Visualization Technique: Body Purification Through Silent Watching

Step 1: Find a quiet place where you will not be disturbed.

Step 2: Sit in a straight-backed chair, with both feet flat on
the floor and your hands facing palms up and resting on
your knees.

Step 3: Close your eyes and inhale and exhale long and
slowly into your lower abdomen (not your chest alone).

Step 4: Listen to the sounds around you. Don't try to focus
on anything in particular.

Step 5: Every few minutes take a long slow deep breath.

Step 6: Finish this visualization by opening your eyes but
remaining in the same spot without moving. Remain quiet
for a few minutes while continuing to listen to the sounds
around you.

Step 7: Become aware of your surroundings and arise while quietly listening to the sounds around you.

*Menu Plan*

**Day 18**

| | |
|---|---|
| Upon Rising | *16-oz. Juice Cocktail #6\** |
| Midmorning | *1 cup vegetable broth* |
| Noontime | *1 bowl of Spicy Garden Vegetable Soup\** |
| Evening | *1 cup Purification Tea with a small amount of honey, if desired* |
| Before Retiring | *1 bowl of miso soup* |

## General Tension-Release Techniques

Try these techniques to release stress through exercising:

1. Clench fists as tightly as possible for about 5 seconds, then release them. Now shake your hands loosely.
2. To relieve headaches and tension around the forehead, raise and lower your eyes as wide as you can, and then squeeze them together as tight as you can. Repeat this process three or four times throughout the day.
4. Perform some range-of-motion exercises. This involves taking each joint in your body; neck, shoulders, elbows, wrists, fingers, hips, knees, ankles. and toes and moving them around clockwise and then counterclockwise.
5. Walk briskly or swim laps for one-half hour three times a week.
6. Use an exercise videotape as you perform aerobic exercise indoors. If you prefer, use a trampoline or other form of rebounding apparatus.
7. *Perform a stress-releasing exercise:* Raise both of your arms over your head and clench your fists tightly. Then hit the bed or the pillow with your forearms and fists at the same time. It's great for releasing your emotional frustrations.

*Menu Plan*

**DAY 19**

Upon Rising                 *16-oz. Juice Cocktail #12\**

Midmorning                  *1 cup Purification Tea with a small amount of honey, if desired.*

Noontime                    *1 bowl of Spicy Garden Vegetable Soup\**

Evening                     *1 cup Purification Tea with a small amount of honey, if desired*

Before                      *16-oz. Juice Cocktail #20\**
Retiring

## Fire Breath

To stimulate your circulation, open blocked sinuses, and increase energy, perform this exercise.

1. Sit on a pad or exercise mat on the floor. Cross your legs "Native American style," forearms over knees, palms up and open, head, neck, and trunk in a straight line.
2. Inhale through your nose into your lower abdomen.
3. Exhale quickly and forcibly by contracting the abdominal muscles.
4. Release the abdominal muscles by a short quick inhalation through your nose.
5. Alternate 10 Fire Breaths with 1 long deep breath three times. That's 30 breaths of fire and three long deep breaths. Do three rounds. If light-headedness occurs, breathe normally.

At first, place your hands just below your navel to get the feeling of the diaphragm expanding and contracting. Notice that your abdomen moves forward on the inhalation and flattens on exhalation. A rapid succession of forcible expulsions is the characteristic of the Fire Breath. The accent is on the exhalation. The Fire Breath can be done sitting, standing, or in any combination of postures.

*Menu Plan*

### Day 20

| | |
|---|---|
| Upon Rising | *16-oz. Juice Cocktail #19* |
| Midmorning | *1 cup Purification Tea with small amount of honey, if desired.* |
| Noontime | *1 bowl of Spicy Garden Vegetable Soup** |
| Evening | *1 cup Purification Tea with a small amount of honey, if desired.* |
| Before Retiring | *1 cup vegetable broth* |

## Side Bend

This yoga-based stretching and strengthening exercise bends your spine laterally while strengthening your lateral torso and hip muscles.

1. Stand with your feet 6 inches apart, with your hands resting lightly on your thighs.
2. Bend sideways from your waist leaning to the right.
3. As you bend to the right, use your right hand as a guide sliding it down your right thigh. Exhale as you bend down, inhale as you come back up to center.
4. Without stopping at the center, bend down sideways to the left, using your left hand as a guide. Exhale as you bend down, inhale as you come up.

Start with 10 bends per side, and add 5 each week until you are doing 25 per side. Make sure the exact line of the exercise is lateral, not forward or backward.

*Menu Plan*

### Day 21

| | |
|---|---|
| Upon Rising | *16-oz. Juice Cocktail #23* |
| Midmorning | *1 cup Purification Tea with a small amount of honey, if desired* |

Noontime                    *1 bowl of Spicy Garden Vegetable Soup**

Evening                     *16-oz. Juice Cocktail #12**

Before                      *1 bowl of miso soup*
Retiring

## Body Shake

This exercise helps to loosen all the muscles in your body.

1. Stand tall.
2. Starting with your feet, shake each part of your body.
3. Repeat this from joint to joint: ankles, knees, waist, shoulders, arms, hand, neck, and head.
4. When you complete each joint, shake your entire body for 5 to 10 seconds.

# SUGGESTED GROCERY LIST FOR WEEK 3

*Fresh Vegetables*: Onion, celery, green pepper, carrot, cucumber, beet, spinach, turnip leaves, watercress, cabbage, medium tomatoes

*Spices (Dried)*: Cayenne pepper powder, bay leaf, onion powder, garlic powder, dried parsley or soup herbs

Prepared miso soup or, if making from scratch, miso paste and distilled water

Whole natural sunflower seeds

Fresh Herbs: Parsley, fresh basil, fresh oregano

Apple

Almond oil, extra-virgin olive oil

Vegebase or vegetable powder

Whole grain alphabet pasta

Distilled water

Soy sauce

Purification tea, honey (optional) for everyday use

# WEEK #4
# REBUILDING YOUR NEW HEALTHY BODY

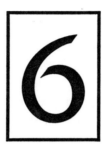

## HOW TO COMBAT A TOXIC ENVIRONMENT WITH SUPER NUTRITION

Everything in our environment is slightly radioactive. Our soil, our food, our water and bodies all contain trace amounts of naturally occurring radioactive isotopes. The majority of these background radioactive particles are soluble in water and thus enter the body, which is more than 90% water. Most of this radioactivity is quickly excreted, resulting in no long-term internal buildup of radioactive isotopes. If you smoke, however, you have a problem that non-smokers avoid. Tobacco contains trace levels of radioactivity, some of which don't wash out of the lungs. These radioactive particles accumulate there and bombard delicate lung tissue with low-level alpha radiation, the same kind of radiation emitted by plutonium.

There are many other herbal and nutritional approaches to cleansing the system of toxic metals and metabolic and other undesirable wastes than those we have already discussed. The ingredients listed here may be placed in a blender filled with fresh apple or papaya juice or, if you wish, ginger or red clover tea.

- *Garlic* is one of nature's better antibiotics. It is useful for treating both bacterial and viral infections. In herbal medicine, chaparral is used for its antiseptic and antibiotic properties. It also works as an "alterative" herb that affects organ and glandular function. This herb helps stimulate and improve the body's blood purification and detoxification.

- *Bee pollen, nutritional yeast, and chlorella (a type of sea algae)* are rich in nucleic acids—an important group of organic substances found especially in the nuclei of all living cells. Nucleic acids are essential to life, and two of the most important nucleic acids, ribonucleic acid (RNA) and deoxyribonucleic acid (DNA)—are crucial to the transmission of hereditary patterns.

- *Onions* contain RNA. Nucleic acids or DNA and RNA are now also sold in the supplement form at some health food stores. There are no established RDAs for nucleic acids.

- *Pectin* has powerful detoxifying qualities and lowers cholesterol.

- *Sodium alginate* absorbs toxins.

- *Flaxseed* is high fiber and is healing to the colon.

- *Psyllium seed* increases bile acid secretion and supplies bulk.

- *Beet root powder* helps to loosen the mucous buildup from the colon walls.

- *Papaya enzyme* helps to digest some of the waste matter that may remain in the stomach.

- *Bentonite* is a natural clay well known among healers for its ability to absorb toxins.

- *Liquid chlorophyll* Increases mineral absorption and helps to reestablish health building bacteria in the system.

### Ten Reasons Why Nutritional Supplementation Is Highly Recommended

1. If you smoke.
2. If you use birth control pills.
3. If you drink alcohol on a regular basis. Alcohol destroys Vitamin $B_2$ and $B_6$, folic acid, and vitamins A, C, and D; it also flushes minerals out of the system.

4. If you drink and smoke at the same time. A combination of vitamin C, vitamin B1, and the amino acid cysteine will assist your body in dealing with the toxic substances produced by these undesirable habits.

5. If you have a food intolerance or sensitivity reactions.

6. If you are on a calorie-restricted diet.

7. If you are avoiding certain foods to reduce your fat intake.

8. If you have poor dietary habits, malabsorption, or past nutritional deficiencies.

9. If you are under considerable physical or emotional stress. Stress can use up large amounts of dietary nutrients, as well as the body's store of vital enzymes and other biochemicals.

10. If you are facing a major medical stress, such as serious burns, major surgery or cancer.

PREVENT KIDNEY STONES AND GALLSTONES WITH LECITHIN

*David R. was a 40-year-old school teacher. He had watched over the years as most of his family went to the hospital for treatment of kidney and gallstones, and was fearful that he would be plagued like most of his other family members. Interested in remaining healthy throughout his life, he began a health maintenance program in his early twenties that included drinking plenty of cleansing juices and using my Liver Flush formula. He also kept his diet low in fats and took lecithin granules daily. Fasting one day a week and exercising regularly, David R. has remained stone free to this day.*

## LECITHIN—NATURE'S PROTECTOR

One of the most important groups of nutrients for body purification are the phospholipids. Probably, the most familiar type of phospholipid is lecithin. Lecithin is a phosphorus-containing fatty compound found in small amounts in most edible plants and was first isolated from egg yolks. The name lecithin is actually derived from the Greek word for this food. Though eggs were the first known source of this nutrient, most of the lecithin found in health food stores and as an added ingredient in various food products is derived from soybeans because soy beans are the least expensive commercial source.

The lecithin in soybeans is particularly rich in both essential fatty acids (linoleic and linoleic), whereas the lecithin found in other foods contains linoleic acid but is low or lacking in linoleic acid. Other nonanimal sources of lecithin include oatmeal, wheat, peanuts, and rice oils.

Many disorders of the brain as well as nervous and muscular disorders may result from exposure to radiation or toxic chemicals. Lecithin may play an important role in protecting the body from these disorders by its important role in the structure of cell membranes in the body. In addition to this, lecithin

- Protects the body against the effects of strontium-90, X-rays, and many other forms of radiation.
- Acts as an antioxidant protecting against radiation and chemical pollutants, including the many consumer devices that emit radiation.
- Protects the body from many common environmental contaminants, including lead, mercury, aluminum, DDT, nitrates, nitrites, and the toxic side effects of many drugs.
- Helps to emulsify and regulate blood cholesterol.
- Aids in the movement of fats across the walls of cells, thus helping to prevent the fatty hardening of arteries.
- Protects the liver and kidneys (key organs for detoxification) and the heart.
- Prevents and dissolves kidney stones and gallstones by emulsifying the fatty substances that can contribute to their formation.
- Is an essential component of bile, where it emulsifies food fats, increasing their surface area and making fat digestion easier through enzymatic action.
- Increases immunity against viral infections, which can be caused by exposure to toxins.
- Increases high-density lipoproteins (the so-called "good"cholesterol, which can lower blood cholesterol), thus protecting the cardiovascular system.
- Assists the detoxifying functions of the liver.
- Increases resistance to disease by its influence on the thymus gland.
- As a phosphatide, is involved in the prevention of cardiovascular problems and atherosclerosis.

- Keeps cholesterol and fats soluble in the blood and prevents them from forming on arterial walls.

## FOUR ANTI-OXIDANTS FOR A LONG AND HEALTHY LIFE

As essential as oxygen is to life, it can also be damaging because of oxidation. This is another reason for using nutritional supplements. Oxidation is the process of oxygen combining with other compounds in our bodies. An example of undesirable oxidation is the interaction oxygen has with components of the cell membrane called lipids. This oxidation reaction results in the breakdown of body cells. The oxidation of lipids also creates peroxides which are damaging to proteins. Lipid peroxidation and damage to crucial proteins causes cells to deteriorate; this is a key component of the aging process. Certain nutrients called antioxidants can reduce the negative effects of oxidation by reducing or stopping oxidation in the body, in those places where it may be harmful.

*The four important antioxidants are*

1. Selenium
2. Superoxide dismutase
3. Vitamins A, C, and E
4. Lecithin

### How Vitamin E, Selenium and Cysteine Got Rid of a Nurse's Arthritis Pain for Good

*A physician in New York related to me the following incident: He had been seeing an elderly nurse as a client for many years. She was plagued by joint pain and swelling. He had prescribed aspirin, gold injections, and even mustard plasters to help reduce her suffering. Unfortunately nothing seemed to work. One day he read an article in a health magazine about how free radicals, little cellular troublemakers, could aggravate arthritis symptoms. He knew that a group of nutrients called antioxidants had the ability to eliminate free radicals from the body. What would happen if he prescribed these? His patient was sent to the health food store where she purchased an antioxidant formula containing the mineral selenium, vitamin E, and the amino acid cysteine. Miraculously after using this formula for only a month, her symptoms had greatly improved.*

# FOOD COMBINING EXPLAINED: NATURAL HYGIENE VERSUS MACROBIOTICS

If you were to listen in on a conversation between any two nutritionists, you would inevitably hear about food combining. There are so many different ideas and myths on the subject that students of nutrition and natural healing often become confused early in their investigations.

There are many theories. While some people advise against eating starch and protein together, others say that eating grains and beans together is the most efficient way of obtaining complete, high-quality protein. Orthodox dietitians say the best food combining plan is the one based on the "four food groups" we learned about in school. This program says that a balanced diet results from eating daily from the meat group, the milk group, the bread and cereal group and the vegetable and fruit group. However, among natural food enthusiasts and those interested in holistic living, the most common food-combining theories are based on the natural hygiene theory and macrobiotics.

## NATURAL HEALING THROUGH NATURAL HYGIENE

Nutrition research has shown that the body can adjust the enzymes and fluids it manufactures for digesting different types of food. There is some evidence that those of us that have weak digestions or suffer from excess stress and tension do not respond well to the combining of many different foods at the same meal. According to some nutritionists, the mixing of many different foods at the same meal will tax the body's enzymatic limitations.

Some of the earliest writings on the subject of food combining were by Sylvester Graham and Doctors Russell Trall, John Tildon, and Herbert Shelton. These men espoused the theory now known as Natural Hygiene, or Life Science. More recently, a best-selling book, *The Fit for Life Diet* by Harvey and Marilyn Diamond, gave these beliefs a popular following. Hygienists believe that certain foods are naturally suited for certain species and that many health problems are caused by straying from the correct eating patterns. According to Shelton, "It is possible to suit the juices to a food, however complex it may be, but not a variety of foods taken together. It is one thing to eat a food; it is quite another to each a complex meal."

According to the philosophy of natural hygiene, poor food combining leads to nutritional deficiencies, the buildup of toxic matter and digestive wastes (resulting from the fermentation of starches and sugars), and the improper digestion of proteins and fats. Simply put, poor food combining leads to poor health.

### Four Guidelines to Apply a Natural Hygienic Approach to Food Combining

1. Avoid eating starchy foods (carrots, potatoes, squash) and acid foods (tomatoes, citrus, etc.) at the same time because the starch-digesting enzymes of the mouth are destroyed by mild acid.

2. Avoid eating sugary foods (most fruits, honey, and other sweeteners) with starchy foods, since the slower digestion of the starches will cause the sugars to be held in the stomach and ferment. Avoid eating honey, maple syrup, barley malt syrup, and jams and jellies with foods such as grains or potatoes. In other words, forget peanut butter and jelly sandwiches.

3. Avoid eating starches and protein foods together. The acidic gastric juices used to digest protein also destroy ptyalin and subsequently stops starch digestion.

4. Protein foods (beans, cheese, animal proteins, such as meat, fish, eggs or poultry) should never be eaten with acid foods, sweet foods, or fats or oils (coconuts, avocados, or any vegetable oils, butter, or margarine). All these foods limit the secretion of gastric juice, and thus delay protein digestion.

## A MACROBIOTIC APPROACH TO FOOD COMBINING:

In macrobiotics foods are seen as contractive for the body (yin) or expansive (yang). The goal is to balance the yin/yang forces. This is done through a form of food combining as described below.

1. At least 50 percent of each meal's volume should consist of whole grains (brown rice, whole barley, millet, kasha).

2. About 5 percent of daily food intake should include a soup consisting of a variety of sea vegetables (arame, wakame, dulse, kelp, hijiki), beans, vegetables, and grains. It is valu-

able to add miso (fermented soybean paste) or tamari soy
sauce to the soup.

3. Approximately 20-30 percent of each meal should include
   vegetables and one-third of the time they should be eaten
   raw. It is best to use foods grown in your area and while
   they are in season.

4. Ten to 15 percent of your food intake should include beans
   and seaweed. Among the most popular beans are black
   beans, aduki, lentils, and chick peas. Seaweeds include nori,
   dulse, wakame, hijiki, and kombu. Moderate amounts of
   tamari soy sauce or sea salt may be used in flavoring.

5. Beverages can include any variety of teas or grain drinks,
   including grain tea. Special macrobiotic teas, such as Mu tea
   or Bancha tea are available at your local health food store.

Many people find that one or the other of these food-combining systems works best for them. Experiment with each and see which is
best for you.

The natural hygiene system is best for those with extremely
weak digestions and for those comfortable in very hot climates. This
is due to the fact that proper food combining is easier on the digestive system. My personal experience has shown that a synthesis of
macrobiotics (grains, beans, salads) combined with a cleansing lactovegetarian diet (fruits, vegetables, nuts, seeds, grains, and fermented dairy products) is the easiest for most people to use.

How a Mother Used Macrobiotics to Magically
Realign Her Life

*Roni S. had tried one diet after another with limited results.
Plagued by arthritis, headaches, fatigue, and multiple colds every
winter, she had almost lost hope of ever being healthy. Roni S.
was constantly trying all kinds of fad diets with little or no result
and denying herself her favorite foods was tortuous.*

*Wanting to save some money so she could take a trip to a spa
Roni began using more beans, grains, low-fat tofu, and other
macrobiotic foods while cutting out heavy expensive meat foods.
Living on root vegetables like carrots, squash, as well as beans
and whole grains, Roni S. discovered that in only 3 days of this
program she began to feel healthier. After 30 days her "stubborn
health problems" had succumbed to the healing powers of macrobiotics. By the the time she was ready to go to the spa she not*

*only had regained her health but shed excess weight as well. She would now have a rice cream breakfast, rice and beans for lunch, and cooked vegetables, including squash, for dinner. For between-meal snacks, she would munch on rice cakes.*

*Macrobiotics helped her regain her health fast and permanently!*

## THE HEALING POWER OF HERBS AND SPICES

Herbs and spices are a cornucopia of nature's gifts. They can heal in many different ways and can be prepared fresh, sprouted, cooked, and even juiced.

Plants have a naturally cleansing and detoxifying effect on the body and mind. They purify the blood and all the tissues of the body, neutralize the waste products of metabolism, and help in building new tissue.

The favorable effect of herbs and spices in the treatment of disease, particularly in combination with juicing, is attributed to the following physiological facts:

- Herbs and spices are extremely rich in vitamins, minerals, trace elements, enzymes, and natural sugars.
- Almost 100% of the vital nutritive elements in juices are assimilated directly from the stomach into the bloodstream, without putting a strain on the digestive system.
- Herbs and spices speed the recovery from disease by supplying needed substances for the body's own healing activity and cell regeneration.
- Fresh herbs and spices provide an alkaline surplus that is extremely important for normalizing the acid-alkaline ration in the blood and tissues, since overacidity is present in most conditions of ill health and is considered to be a contributing factor in disease development.
- Generous amounts of easily assimilable organic minerals in herbs and spices, particularly calcium, potassium, and silicon, help to restore biochemical and mineral balance in the tissues and cells. Mineral imbalance in the tissues is one of the main causes of diminished oxygenation, which leads to premature aging of cells and disease.

- Herbs, spices, and different vegetables contain nature's own medicines, vegetable hormones, and antibiotics. For example, string beans are known to contain insulinlike substances; cucumbers and onions contain hormones needed by the cells of the pancreas to produce insulin; and antibiotic substances are present in fresh garlic, onions, radishes, and tomatoes.
- Studies show that raw herbs, fruits, and vegetables contain, as yet, an unidentified factor that is responsible for the cells' ability to absorb nutrients from the bloodstream and effectively excrete metabolic wastes from the cell.
- The various coloring substances, red, yellow, green, and blue, in all shades and intensities, which are present in fruits, vegetables, and herbs, are vitally important from a therapeutic point of view. They increase production of red blood corpuscles, influence digestive and assimilative processes, and take part in the metabolism of proteins and cholesterol.

It is easy to see, then, why herbs, spices, nuts, seeds, grains, fruits, and vegetables have such an important role to play in the 30-Day Body Purification Program.

## Mullein

This herb is a wonderful healer for the lungs, and lung ailments such as asthma, bronchitis, and clogged sinuses. The lungs are an important organ of elimination and mullein is effective in making respiration more efficient, which is essential in the detoxification-purification process.

## Golden Seal

Golden seal is a yellow root, first used by the Cherokee Indians as a blood purifier. Its tonifying qualities are most commonly used for the kidneys and liver, thus helping these organs to eliminate toxic substances, including nicotine and opiates, from the bloodstream and body. This herb is extremely bitter and, for this reason, is frequently ingested in capsules. Sometimes, it is mixed into capsules with another powdered herbal stimulant, cayenne pepper, as a tonic for the digestive and circulatory systems.

One of the best herbs for internal purification, golden seal is the strongest of the natural antibiotics. Even so, it should be used in moderation. Though this herb has been shown to kill various types of bacteria, large doses of golden seal will probably also kill some of the helpful bacteria in the intestines. Therefore, eating a dish of yogurt or drinking kefir with acidophilus culture will help restore the necessary balance of bacteria in the intestinal tract if golden seal is consumed regularly.

## Spearmint

Spearmint offers a mild, natural tranquilizing effect. It is calming to the stomach, as well as to the nervous system. It is an aid to digestion, helps to expel gas, and is excellent for various gastric disturbances. Spearmint helps relieve headaches and other symptoms in those trying to give up coffee and tobacco products by allowing them to relax and go to sleep naturally.

Frequently, individuals crave sedating agents because of anxiety and nervousness. A mixture of chamomile and spearmint has been used successfully as a mild sedative.

## Rose Hips

Studies have shown that Vitamin C promotes healing and detoxification of bodily poisons. Rose hips are one of the best natural sources of Vitamin C. Vitamin C protects against toxic chemicals in the environment, relieves physical and emotional stress, prevents the common cold, and helps strengthen the heart, teeth, and bones.

Rose hips are added to the Purification Tea as much for their delicious fruity taste as for their healing qualities. Rose hips are the natural fruit of the rose bush; they form after the petals fall off. They look like small red berries and are very high in various nutrients, including Vitamins A, C, E, $B_{12}$, and K, bioflavinoids, calcium, iron, and phosphorous.

Bioflavinoids (or Vitamin P) are needed for the proper absorption and use of Vitamin C. In addition, Vitamin P is useful in hypertension and respiratory infection.

## Orange Peel

Similarly, orange peel contains a good amount of Vitamin C and bioflavinoids, as well as having a great taste. However, make sure that whatever orange peels you use in the Purification Tea, they are organic and have not been sprayed with insecticides or herbicides.

Cinnamon powder, a popular spice made from the leaves and bark of the tree, is used primarily for flavoring cakes, puddings, bread, buns, and stewed fruits. It was popular for many years as a light tea for upset stomachs. Cinnamon, when mixed with apple pectin or grated apple skins, will slow down and even stop diarrhea. Cinnamon Tea for Upset Stomach

Add 1/2 teaspoon of cinnamon powder to 6 oz. of boiling distilled water. Let it sit for about 10 minutes and steep slowly.

## Garlic

Garlic has been used as a medicinal herb since antiquity. In the Middle Ages, it was used as a cure for worms and even leprosy. In recent years, it has become popular as a natural antibiotic and is commonly used in treating infections, colds, and influenza. Due to its high sulphur, many people find that it has a mild tranquilizing effect. It was always believed to increase circulation, and recent medical studies indicate that it can actually reduce high blood pressure and cholesterol.

*Formula for Garlic Oil*

8 oz. of peeled or minced garlic

4 oz. of warm extra virgin-olive oil, sufficient to cover the garlic

## Siberian Ginseng

This herb (Eleuthero or Eleutherococcus senticosus) is called Siberian ginseng because it is native to parts of China and Russia. As a fluid extract, Eleuthero, possesses many healing and purifying properties, including

Protecting the body against stress, various chemical toxins, and environmental pollutants;

Offering radioactivity protection. It can be used therapeutically in conditions of acute and chronic radiation sickness, such as hemorrhaging, severe anemia, dizziness, nausea, vomiting, and headaches due to X rays. If you are receiving X rays or radiation treatments, use Eleuthero extract.

Neutralizing the ill effects caused by drugs and other substances.

Counteracting some of the side effects of cortisone treatment, such as adverse changes in the weight of the adrenals.

Significantly improving human immune response.

Preventing harmful effects of stress, such as stomach bleeding, and disrupted production of adrenaline.

Aiding in the absorption and retention of some important protective nutrients, including Vitamins $B_1$ and $B_2$ and Vitamin C.

There is no combination of herbs and foods more protective against radiation and environmental pollutants than Siberian ginseng and sea vegetables.

### HOW AN ALREADY HEALTHY ATHLETE FOUND INCREASED ENERGY, HAD FEWER COLDS, AND NEEDED LESS SLEEP AFTER TAKING SIBERIAN GINSENG

*Neil M. eats well, and he exercises regularly. However, he has a great deal of emotional stress, and he has various allergic nose and throat disorders that weaken his immunity to colds. The resulting colds aren't minor either. Whenever Neil catches a cold, he has a rough hacking cough at night, a runny nose, and constant congestion all day. This interferes with his jogging schedule and leaves him tired and depleted of all energy.*

*One day, a friend mentioned that he to had been plagued with colds but they had stopped when he began using an herb called Siberian ginseng. Though not actually the same as regular "ginseng," he related, this herb had been shown to have many of the health building qualities as the more popular Chinese variety. Neil began following a specific program for preventing and treating colds that included Siberian ginseng:*

1. At the first sign of a cold, Neil saw to it that he got 2 or 3 days of bed rest and    followed a proper diet. He increased his intake of warm fluids to maintain body fluids and loosen mucous.

2. He avoided stress.

3. He used steam with essence of eucalyptus or essence of thyme to expectorate mucus, and he lubricated his nostrils with a comfrey salve to reduce irritation.

4. To reduce pain, inflammation, and fever, Neil used white willow bark tablets, which contain salicin, a natural substance that is related to aspirin.

5. He supplemented his diet with vitamins A and C.

6. Neil eliminated immune-depressing stimulants, such as alcohol, tobacco, coffee, tea, chocolate and sugar.

7. To prevent cracking of the nasal mucous membranes, he used a humidifier to offset the effects of heat in his apartment.

8. He began using herbal teas and following juice therapy formulas with plenty of carrot and citrus juices. He also went through a general internal detoxification program.

9. As his symptoms changed, he used whichever homeopathic remedies were appropriate.

Following the program, Neil can now effectively stop the full symptoms of a cold from setting in by following a natural healing approach. His "colds" typically last for only a day or 2—rarely more than 3 days—as compared with the 14-day colds he once had.
But most of all, his energy level has greatly increased. This he attributes to Siberian ginseng.

## WEEK 4: DAILY MENU PLANS, EXERCISES, AND MEDITATIONS

Week #4 gives you the opportunity to build the foundation of your nutritional program for the future. The menus for the next seven days are rich in herbs and spices, which are not only flavorful but filled with essential nutrients.

If you are coming off of a week of fasting avoid excessive use of grains, beans, and dairy products, which are heavier on the digestive processes. Focus more on juicing and eating fresh fruit and vegetable salads.

In addition to a regular natural multiple vitamin-mineral supplement, take an antioxidant supplement daily. Antioxidant supplements can be obtained in your local health food store.

## Menu Plan

### Day 22

Breakfast

*16 oz. Juice Formula #3\**
*1 cup fresh fruit salad — oranges, grapefruit,*
*tangerine*
*Herbal tea or coffee substitute*

Lunch

*1 bowl of miso soup*
*1/2 cup brown rice with Tomato Sauce\**
*1/2 cup tofu*
*1 cup of a steamed, pleasant-tasting sea veg-*
*etable (arame, wakamae, kombu, hijiki, nori)*
*1/2 cup steamed carrots*
*1 ear corn on the cob*

Dinner

*6 oz. Herbed Tofu Pilaf\**
*1 cup chopped cucumber*
*1 medium tomato, sliced*
*1 cup romaine lettuce*
*1 cup of a steamed, pleasant-tasting sea veg-*
*etable (arame, wakamae, kombu, hijiki, nori)*
*1 medium apple*
*Herbal tea or coffee substitute*

## Body Stretch

In addition to strengthening the Achilles tendon hamstring, heart, and shoulders, this exercise is also valuable for those suffering from sleep disorders.

1. Stand tall.
2. Raise your hands above your head.
3. Now stretch your arms and fingers as if you are reaching for the stars and clawing the air.
4. As you reach, inhale deeply through your nostrils while rising on your toes.

---

\* Recipes for starred beverages, main dishes, soups, and sauces may be found in Appendix IV, "Herbs and Spices," Appendix V, "Your Home Guide to Juicing," and Appendix VII, "Purification Recipes."

5. Exhale slowly, and gradually return to the starting position, with your arms hanging loosely at your side.
6. Repeat this at least three times.

*Menu Plan*

**Day 23**

Breakfast
*16 oz. Juice Formula #3\**
*1 cup fresh pineapple*
*Herbal tea or coffee substitute*

Lunch
*6 oz. Spicy Mushroom-Sage Stuffing*
*1 cup of a steamed, pleasant-tasting sea vegetable (arame, wakamae, kombu, hijiki, nori)*
*2 cups romaine lettuce*
*8 oz. nonfat yogurt (plain or flavored)*
*Choice of beverage*

Dinner
*6 oz. Pine Nut Tabbouleh*
*1 cup chopped cucumber*
*1 medium tomato, sliced*
*1 cup romaine lettuce*
*1 medium pear*
*Herbal tea or coffee substitute*

## Yoga Head/Neck Release

According to yoga experts, this exercise helps relieve headache and stimulates metabolism.

1. Standing, with your feet 6 inches apart, arms by sides, drop your chin to your chest.
2. Press chin lightly on chest, then move right ear toward the right shoulder and then the left ear toward the left shoulder.
3. Repeat step 2 to the left three times.

Relax your shoulders, and with your eyes closed, focus on the point between your eyebrows. Take long and deep breaths. Remember to roll your head slowly.

*Menu Plan*

**DAY 24**

Breakfast
: *16 oz. Juice Formula #3\**
*1 cup tropical fresh fruit salad—banana, mango, papaya*
*Herbal tea or coffee substitute*

Lunch
: *1 bowl of E-Z ABC Soup\**
*6 oz. Herbed Tofu Pilaf\**
*1 cup of a steamed, pleasant-tasting sea vegetable (arame, wakamae, kombu, hijiki, nori)*
*1/2 cup steamed pumpkin*
*1 cup steamed cauliflower*

Dinner
: *6 oz. Tempeh Salad\**
*1 cup of a steamed, pleasant-tasting sea vegetable (arame, wakamae, kombu, hijiki, nori)*
*1 cup chopped cucumber*
*1 medium tomato, sliced*
*1 cup romaine lettuce (Sweet Dill Dressing\*)*
*8 oz. nonfat yogurt (plain or flavored)*
*Herbal tea or coffee substitute*

## Body Bend

This is a classic exercise for releasing tight hamstring muscles.

1. Stand tall.
2. Slowly bend from the waist, loosely dropping your head and arms. Do not bounce or force the stretch. Let it come naturally.
3. Inhale slowly through your mouth. (This will automatically lift your torso.)
4. Exhale slowly. (This will automatically lower your torso and bring your fingers closer to your toes.)
5. Inhale and exhale three times.

*Menu Plan*

**Day 25**

Breakfast                    *16 oz. Juice Formula #1\**
*1/2 cup nonfat, fruit juice-sweetened granola*
*Herbal tea or coffee substitute*

Lunch                        *6 oz. Tempeh Salad\**
*1 cup of a steamed, pleasant-tasting sea veg-*
*etable (arame, wakamae, kombu, hijiki,*
*nori)*
*1 cup chopped cucumber*
*1 medium tomato, sliced*
*1 cup romaine lettuce (Choice of Spa*
*Dressing)*
*Tofu Protein Pops\**
*Herbal tea or coffee substitute*

Dinner                       *6 oz. Mock Chicken Salad*
*3/4 cup mashed potatoes with garlic and*
*extra virgin olive oil*
*1 medium tomato, sliced*
*2 cups romaine lettuce (choice of Spa*
*Dressing\*)*

## Cradle Stretch

This exercise will strengthen your lower back and abdominal muscles.

1. Lie flat on your back
2. Bend your knees and slowly bring them to your chest, with your arms folded around them.
3. As you draw your knees to your chest, inhale deeply.
4. Now exhale, and as you do so, draw your legs even closer to your chest.
5. Inhale and exhale three times.
6. Slowly straighten your legs and lower them to the floor.

Start with 10 of these; add 10 a week until you reach 50. Remember to keep elbows up at shoulder level.

*Menu Plan*

### Day 26

Breakfast

*16 oz. Juice Formula #3*
*1 cup fresh fruit salad—oranges, grapefruit, tangerines*
*Herbal tea or coffee substitute*

Lunch

*6 oz. Tofu Vegetable Casserole**
*1/2 cup steamed broccoli*
*1/2 cup steamed cauliflower*
*2 cups romaine lettuce (Ginger Peanut Dressing*)*
*1 serving baked peaches*
*Choice of beverage*

Dinner

*6 oz. Spicy Mushroom-Sage Stuffing**
*1 cup of a steamed, pleasant-tasting sea vegetables (arame, wakamae, kombu, hijiki, nori)*
*2 cups romaine lettuce*
*Pear and Apple Compote**
*Choice of beverage*

## Leg Lift

This exercise is great for toning the abdomen and lower back muscles and for stretching thigh muscles.

1. Lie flat on your back.
2. Lift your legs off the floor about three feet.
3. Inhale deeply as you raise your legs. Hold them in the position described in  step 2 as long as you can while holding your breath.
4. Then exhale slowly while lowering your legs.
5. Perform this exercise three times.

*Menu plan*

### Day 27

Upon Rising          *Juice Cocktail #1**

Lunch                    *1 bowl of miso soup*
                         *1/2 brown rice with tomato sauce*
                         *1/2 cup lentils*
                         *1 cup of a steamed, pleasant-tasting sea veg-*
                         *etable*
                         *(arame, wakamae, kombu, hijiki, nori) with*
                         *Red Garlic Dressing\**
                         *1/2 cup steamed carrots*
                         *1 cup steamed cauliflower*

Dinner                   *1 bowl of Spicy Garden Vegetable Soup\**
                         *1 mixed vegetable salad consisting of*
                         *    1 cup grated carrots*
                         *    1 medium tomato, sliced*
                         *    2 cups romaine lettuce*
                         *    Tart Tahini Dressing\**
                         *Herbal tea or coffee substitute*

## Foot Rotation

Strengthen the toes, foot, and ankle muscles as follows:

1. Stand tall.
2. Lift one foot about 12 inches from the floor.
3. Flex the foot up and down, 6 times in each direction.
4. Rotate the foot, 12 times counterclockwise and 12 times clockwise.
5. Repeat for the other foot.

*Menu Plan*

**Day 28**

Breakfast                *8 oz. freshly squeezed orange juice*
                         *8 oz. nonfat yogurt (vanilla flavored or add*
                         *vanilla extract)*
                         *Herbal tea or coffee substitute*

Lunch                    *1 bowl of Spicy Garden Vegetable Soup\**
                         *1/2 cup kasha*
                         *1/2 cup white beans*

|  | 1 cup of a steamed, pleasant-tasting sea vegetable<br>(arame, wakamae, kombu, hijiki, nori)<br>1/2 cup baked butternut squash<br>1 cup steamed broccoli |
|---|---|
| Dinner | 2 Barley Burgers*<br>1 whole ear of corn on the cob<br>1 cup steamed cauliflower<br>2 cups romaine lettuce (choice of Spa Dressing*)<br>1 serving baked peaches<br>Choice of beverage |

## Aerobic Dancing

This is great for reducing stress and building the cardiovascular system. Play some upbeat music and dance. Dance vigorously for at least five minutes. Be as creative as you can, engaging your whole body, and constantly moving.

## SUGGESTED GROCERY LIST FOR WEEK 4

*Fresh Vegetables:* Celery, cabbage, beet, cucumber, carrots, corn on the cob, scallions, cucumber, medium tomatoes, romaine lettuce (or boston lettuce in some recipes), mushrooms, shallots, pumpkin, cauliflower, celery, radishes, bean sprouts, butternut squash, broccoli, onions

*Fresh Fruit:* Oranges, grapefruits, tangerines, banana, mango, papaya, apple, nectarine or peach, pear, pineapple, lemon (or lime in some recipes), medium pear, medium apple

*Spices:* Dried rosemary, sea salt, white or black peppercorns, dried mint flakes, dried thyme, dried parsley or soup herbs, bay leaves, cayenne pepper powder, garlic powder, dried thyme, dried oregano, dried basil

*Herbs (Fresh):* garlic, fresh basil, fresh parsley, fresh sage, fresh mint leaves, fresh parsley, fresh dill fresh oregano, onion powder, garlic powder

*Sea Vegetables:* Arame, wakamae, kombu, hijiki, nori—one or

as many as desired
Brown rice—short grain, or whatever is available
Extra virgin olive oil, canola oil
Crushed tomatoes
Herbal tea or coffee substitute for everyday use
Miso soup—prepared miso soup or, if making from scratch, miso paste and distilled water
Vegebase or vegetable powder
Distilled water
Bulghur (cracked wheat)
Organically grown lemon rind
Whole natural (unblanched) almonds
Extra-virgin olive oil, canola oil, or almond oil for selected recipes
Seedless raisins or currants
Firm tofu
Nonfat yogurt (plain or flavored)
Choices of beverage
Unroasted pinenuts
Whole grain alphabet pasta
Light soy sauce
Tempeh
Slivered almonds (untoasted), filberts or other nuts
Raw sesame seeds
Apple cider vinegar, red wine vinegar
Dijon mustard
Honey
Nonfat, fruit juice-sweetened granola
Frozen juice concentrate
Pure vanilla extract
Popsicle sticks for tofu protein pops
TVP (textured vegetable protein)
Eggless, low-fat tofu-based mayonnaise
Lentils

White beans
Tahini
Tamari
Kasha
Whole barley or medium pearled barley

# MAINTAINING YOUR HEALTHY BODY

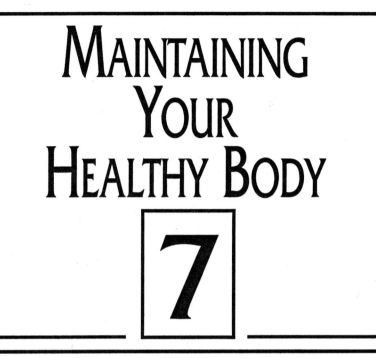

After you have completed the 30-Day Body Purification Program, it is essential to maintain the healthy body you have created. You require over 40 different nutrients. These include amino acids (from proteins), essential fatty acids (from fats and oils), and sources of energy (calories from carbohydrates, fats and proteins). Of course water is essential for good health as well. Vitamins and minerals are also essential.

Each of us has different work schedules, different responses to stress, and likewise our nutritional requirements may be different from those of others. Don't be afraid to experiment with amounts of this or that, until you see what combination of suggestions works best for you. Also, it may be helpful to seek individual consultation to learn more about the most effective diet for your special nutritional needs. Recognize, too, that your nutritional requirements will vary at different times in your life, and at different seasons of the year, and that they are greatly affected by the stress of any significant changes in your life.

To be sure that you are doing all that you can to eat properly and maintain the benefits of the 30-Day Body Purification Program, please keep the following information at hand and use it to guide you. These suggestions will apply to most people; however, if you have a special health problem look it up in the index at the back of the book and adjust your program accordingly.

## GUIDELINES FOR PURIFIED NUTRITION

Many nutritionists still use the four basic food group concept of meal structure. You can use this approach so long as you avoid unhealthy foods and build your lifestyle on a whole foods model. However you eat do so with moderation as a guideline. Eating sensible amounts of a variety of foods makes for a nutritionally balanced diet, helps you enjoy your meals, and can help keep calories—and weight—under control. Notice that sweets and desserts are not included; servings of these foods should be limited since these foods generally contain few vitamins and minerals.

Choosing a variety of foods means staying away from fad diets—for example, an "all protein"diet or an "all apples" diet. In recommending large amounts of certain foods, some diets lack the balance and variety essential to good nutrition and long-term weight control. They may even pose a health risk by depriving your body of essential nutrients. The following general guidelines are suggested for those who have completed the 30-Day Body Purification Program and would like to maintain good health.

### The Five Basic Food Groups for Body Purification

1. Fats, oils
2. Bean and grain combinations
3. Nuts and seeds (two servings a day)
3. Vegetables and fruit
5. Dairy products

## NINE TIPS TO KEEP YOUR PURIFICATION PROGRAM ON TRACK

1. Eat a variety of fresh, unrefined, and unprocessed foods, especially fresh fruits and vegetables, whole grain breads, cereals, pasta and other whole grain products, yogurt, but-

termilk, skim milk, goat's milk, unprocessed cheeses and other milk products, dry beans and peas. (Note: Dairy products should be limited if you suffer from respiratory complaints.)

2. Avoid most canned vegetables and fruits. There are a few brands of organically grown foods in cans but these are generally available only in health food stores. Whenever possible buy fruits, vegetables, nuts, seeds, grains, and beans that have been produced without the use of pesticides and commercial fertilizer. If you do not have access to organically grown produce, health food stores carry products that can wash off pesticides from the fruit and vegetable skin. Sprouting is another option.

3. Read labels carefully to determine how much processing and what type of additives have been put in the food. Some additives and residues have been statistically associated with a number of major diseases and disabilities.

4. Add complex carbohydrates to your meals while decreasing your intake of other foods such as meats and high-fat dairy products. Complex carbohydrate foods are generally less expensive than these foods and are good sources of vitamins and minerals. You'll also benefit from a lower intake of saturated fats and cholesterol.

5. Shake the salt habit. Learn to enjoy the natural taste of foods by reducing your use of iodized salt, sea salt, and soy sauce in cooking and by removing it from the table.

6. Avoid or severely limit your use of stimulants or depressants. They offer little or nothing nutritionally and can inhibit and even damage the nervous system. This would include alcoholic beverages, coffee, pekoe teas, tobacco, chocolate, and black and white pepper.

7. Avoid or severely limit your use of all fried foods and artificially colored, flavored or preserved snack foods (potato, corn and cheese chips, and the like).

8. Avoid or severely limit your use of animal products, particularly eggs, meat, and fish, due to the excessive level of pollutants, hormones, and sanitary problems that are associated with them.

9. Beware of foods labeled "Natural." Most commercial yogurt products contain unacceptable additives, and along with most commercial ice creams contain refined sugar.

# FOODS TO INCLUDE/FOODS TO AVOID

## Bread Baked at Home

*Include*: Natural yeasts, living starters, unleavened products.
*Avoid*: Baking powder, baking soda, preserved yeast.

## Beverages

*Include*: Herb teas—chamomile, mint, papaya—fresh fruit juice; fresh vegetable juice.
*Avoid*: Alcohol, caffeine (cocoa, coffee, and carbonated beverages), canned and pasteurized juices, artificial fruit drinks.

## Carbohydrates

*Include*: Whole grain sources of starch and fiber. Whole grains are high in complex carbohydrates and high-quality fiber. The most common varieties are whole wheat, rye, corn, whole unrefined corn meal, barley, buckwheat (kasha), millet, brown rice, 100% whole grain breads, pita pockets, pasta and pancake mixes.
*Avoid*: Refined white flour products, such as white rice, pasta, white flour pita pockets, white bread and other low fiber wheat, and rye and other dark breads that are made from white flour with coloring and preservatives added.

## Cheese

*Include*: White raw cheese, 99% fat-free cottage cheese, Hoop cheese.
*Avoid*: High-fat cheeses and any pasteurized processed cheeses and cheese spreads.

NOTE: *Instead of cream cheese, use Neufchatel cheese and use skimmed or partially skimmed milk cheese (mozzarella, St. Ortho, Jarlsburg, etc.) to reduce your caloric intake.*

## Chocolate

*Include*: Carob and carob powders.
*Avoid*: Chocolate, cocoa, and carob candy bars made from hydrogenated vegetable oil.

## Dairy Products

*Include*: Raw milk, sugar-free low-fat yogurt, butter, and buttermilk in limited quantities; nonfat cottage cheese and white cheese.
*Avoid*: All processed and imitation butter (margarine) any yogurts containing Nutrasweet™, sugar, cane syrup, gelatin, modified food starch, or any artificial colors or flavors.

NOTE: *One food that people are most sensitive to is cow's milk. Reactions may be classical allergic reactions but others are less specific. To respond, for example, to the "threat" of cow's milk, the body sets its defense system into action when this food enters the body. It is not always clear why many people have reactions to cow's milk products. For some, it is a deficiency in a particular enzyme (lactase) that is used by the body to digest milk sugar (lactose). This enzyme deficiency is called lactose intolerance. Some react only to plain cow's milk but not to processed milk products such as butter, yogurt, sour cream, or buttermilk. It is not always readily apparent as to why a person might react to milk, but sometimes they just do.*

## Desserts

*Include*: Fruit-flavored yogurt, fresh fruit compote, or any desserts listed in the recipe section in the back of the book.
*Avoid*: Ice cream.

## Dressings (Salad Dressings and Various Condiment Sauces)

*Include*: Dressings prepared from dried herbs and herb blends, tofu, nonfat yogurt, extra-virgin olive oil, Tabasco sauce, homemade ketchup, homemade barbecue sauce, natural mayonnaise (homemade or natural food store eggless, tofu-based variety).

*Avoid*: Pourable salad dressing (read label for oil content and composition; some may contain coconut or palm oil). Avoid commercially bottled or packaged dressings containing monosodium glutamate (M.S.G.), modified food starch, artificial colors, flavors or preservatives, ketchup with sugar, A-1 sauce, and so on.

NOTE: *In recipes calling for mayonnaise, use low-fat yogurt, buttermilk, or a low-calorie, no-cholesterol mayonnaise substitute that is available in a health food store.*

## Fruits

*Include*: All dried (unsulphured), stewed, fresh, frozen (unsweetened) fruit.
*Avoid*: Canned, sweetened fruit.

## Grains

*Include*: Whole grain sources of starch and fiber. Whole grains are used in certain cereals, breads, and muffins. The most easily available whole grains are rye, oats, wheat, bran, buckwheat, millet, cream of wheat, brown rice, corn, and whole seeds (sesame, pumpkin, sunflower, flaxseed).
*Avoid*: While flour products, hulled grains and seeds (e.g., pasta, crackers, macaroni, snack foods, white rice, prepared or cold cereals, cooked seeds).

## Nuts

*Include*: All fresh, raw nuts, nuts in shell, and blanched and home-roasted whole nuts.

*Avoid*: Roasted, dry-roasted, and/or salted nuts, especially peanuts.

## Fats and Oils

*Include*: Expeller pressed  unsaturated, unrefined oils, (corn, sesame, safflower, extra-virgin olive, soybean, peanut); dressings made from safflower, corn), and eggless mayonnaise,

*Avoid*: Highly processed and chemically refined fats and oils (unsaturated as well as saturated); margarine or any type and mayonnaise; foods high in saturated fats, such as meat drippings, coconut oil, palm kernel oil, hydrogenated and partially hardened vegetable shortenings; foods high in both saturated fats and cholesterol, such as lard, lard-based shortenings, beef fat, beef fat-based shortening, and butter, sour cream and other whole milk- or cream-based dairy  products. Read package labels when choosing processed foods. Remember that "vegetable oil" could mean coconut or palm oil, both high in saturated fat.

NOTE: *Remember which foods  are dietary sources of saturated fats and  cholesterol. As a rule of thumb, saturated fats and cholesterol are generally found in foods from animal sources, while polyunsaturated fats come from vegetable sources— coconut and palm oil are the exceptions.*

## Protein Sources

*Include:* There are many excellent vegetarian proteins.

1. Sunflower seeds or meal, raw, unsalted.
2. Sesame seeds or meal (try the protein-aids brand).
3. Raw, unsalted nuts such as almonds, pignolias, Brazil nuts, or pecans. Ground meal or butters of these nuts are also excellent, but should always be raw and unsalted.
4. Soybeans, garbanzo beans (chick peas). These should be soaked overnight so that they will not require as much cooking. Dried lentils, kidney beans, lima beans, and split peas

are also fine proteins. Beans form an even higher-quality protein when combined with grains such as brown rice, millet, and corn or sesame seeds.

5. Brewer's yeast is also a fine protein source. We recommend brands that are calcium-magnesium balanced.

6. Bee pollen pellets are a fine source of protein and B-vitamins.

7. Bovine hormone—free low-fat milk and other dairy products.

8. Tofu.

9. Tempeh.

10. Green magma.

11. Micro algae—spirulina, chlorella, and so on.

*Avoid:* Meat, fish, poultry, eggs, high-fat dairy products.

## Seasonings

*Include*: Herbs, garlic, onion, parsley, marjoram, cayenne pepper, pure sugar-free extracts. Choose low-sodium seasonings such as lemon or lime juice, herbs, spices, and salt substitute (check with a medical advisor before using). To avoid hidden sodium in foods, choose salt-free bakery goods, fresh fruit, raw vegetables, unsalted nuts, unsalted unbuttered popcorn, fresh or frozen vegetables, and homemade soups.

*Avoid*: Black and white pepper, salt; chemical imitation flavorings; and barbeque or soy sauce with sugar, preservatives, artificial flavors, or colors added. Higher-sodium foods include ketchup, relish, mustard, soy sauce, barbecue sauce, prepared frozen dinners, processed or salted meats, fish and poultry, potato chips, pretzels, salted nuts, salted buttered popcorn, canned vegetables, canned soups, and powered bouillon.

NOTE: *If your medical advisor has given you instructions to decrease sodium and salt intake and increase your potassium, learn which foods—and how much of them—satisfy your potassium needs. Foods high in potassium are oranges, bananas, peanuts, potatoes, and beans. You can also use my Potassium Broth formula.*

## Snack Foods

*Include*: Natural corn munchies, rice cakes, nuts, and seeds.
*Avoid*: Potato chips, corn chips, pretzels (unless whole grain), salted nuts, and salted buttered popcorn.

## Soups

*Include*: Homemade soup (e.g., salt-free vegetable), natural vegetable bouillon from a health food store.
*Avoid*: Canned and creamed (thickened) soups, commercial bouillon, fat stock.

## Sprouts

*Include*: All, especially wheat, pea, lentil, alfalfa, and mung.
*Avoid*: All varieties are acceptable.

## Sweets

*Include*: Raw honey (not to be used by children under 2 years of age), unsulphured molasses, carob, barley malt or rice syrup. Pure maple syrup and Sucanat (dehydrated sugar cane juice) can be used in limited amounts.
Avoid: Foods containing refined sugars (white, brown, turbinado), chocolate, candy, syrups, sugar syrups, and so on; fructose, high-fructose corn syrup; glucose; eating sweets between meals.

*Note: When buying packaged foods read the labels for information on sugar content. Studies have shown refined white sugar to be a source of food sensitivity as well as a factor in tooth decay and a possible factor in various health problems—for instance, low blood sugar (hypoglycemia), elevation of triglyceride levels, which could result in hypertension, and loss of minerals, including calcium from the body.*

*When discussing sugar most people think of table sugar (sucrose), but there are many other types of refined sugar as well. Being familiar with the all the other labels for sugar will be of help when your grocery shopping. They are glucose (dextrose), high fructose corn sweetener, maltose, and lactose.*

- Limit sugary desserts. Instead, top off your meal occasionally with fresh fruits, which both satisfy your desire for sweets and provide valuable nutrients.
- To reduce sugar intake from soft drinks, limit intake or dilute them with seltzer water.
- If you add sugar to foods such as coffee, tea, or cereal, add less each time; you may gradually eliminate it.

## Vegetables

*Include*: Vegetables in season. All raw and not overcooked fresh or frozen, potatoes baked or boiled.
*Avoid:* Packaged, frozen, canned vegetables, fried potatoes in any form.

## COOKING TIPS FOR BODY PURIFICATION

The way food is prepared can be just as important to health and body purification as the food itself. By using cooking techniques such as the ones that follow, you can improve the nutritional value of the foods you eat.

- Try quick steaming or eating vegetables raw. The natural flavors of vegetables are preserved when quick methods of preparation are used.
- Be creative in your cooking. Try adding new flavors to foods, such as lemon or lime juice, onions, garlic, green chiles, horseradish, cayenne pepper, vinegar, or even a "pinch" of honey.

If you are unwilling to cut out meat from your diet, keep the following cooking tips in mind:

- Trim excess fat from meat before cooking.
- Roast and broil foods on a rack so fat can drain off.

- Brown meats and poultry; then pour off fat before you continue cooking.
- Baste meats with tomato juice or a canola oil-vinegar marinade rather than meat drippings.
- Make pot roasts and stews a day ahead. Chill them and scrape off congealed fat; then reheat.
- Use extra-virgin olive oil for pan frying, stir frying, and sauteing, and salad dressings.

## DINING OUT THE HEALTHY WAY

Eating out and staying true to The Body Purification principles is easier than you might think. Here are some tips on how to eat out in any restaurant and be healthy.

1. Ask whether you can get a smaller portion than is usually served. Less food on the plate means fewer calories from the meals.
2. Ask how foods are prepared, especially about the use of salt, butter, and other saturated fats. Knowing what the chef puts into the dish can help you order wisely.
3. Order all dishes without heavy sauces or gravies.
4. Skip the creamy salad dressings; instead ask for oil and vinegar on the side so that you can control the quantity.
5. Share appetizers, entrees, and desserts. Just a taste of a dish can be as satisfying as eating the whole thing!
6. Eat more slowly than you usually do. This can help you recognize when you feel satisfied and prevent overeating. Stop eating before you feel full; what you don't finish can always be taken home.
7. Ask for a dessert of fresh fruit or fruit ice. Your sweet tooth may never know the difference between these and rich, heavy desserts.
8. The way food is prepared can be just as important to health and weight control as the food itself. By using cooking techniques such as steaming or broiling, you can improve the nutritional value of the foods you eat, no matter where you are.

## Exploring Emotional Health

Emotional health is a key factor in creating and maintaining physical health. Review the following questions about emotional health and creating healthy relationships and see how many emotional health patterns and communication skills you currently exhibit.

- Do you acknowledge your own anger?
- Do you listen closely when other express their anger or do you ignore or try to laugh off the anger?
- Do you communicate to others when you are angry?
- When another person is angry do you hurry the person and try to shut them up? Do you give others the opportunity to communicate their anger?
- Do you have a violent temper or do you have the ability to keep calm?
- Do you sometimes say things that you don't really mean?
- Are you able to solve problems before you become overwhelmed with rage?
- When you are dealing with someone else who is very angry, are you able to encourage them to talk about solving the problem that caused the anger?
- When dealing with an angry person, do you have the ability to talk reasonably with the person, propose a specific solution to the problem, and agree on a schedule to implement the solution?
- Are you involved in small group activities and service organizations?
- Are you a loner, or do you support other people's efforts to go beyond the limitations of fear?
- Are you involved in creating healthy relationships with friends and family?
- Are you able to ask family and friends for support when you require it?
- Do you offer family and friends emotional support when they are in need, whether or not they are willing to accept it?
- Do you choose your circumstances and environment for work and play consciously?

- Do you believe that a creative work environment is important for emotional health?
- Do you sit watching anything that appears on the television screen?
- Do you look to expand your interests, try new things, or do you do things merely out of habit?
- Do you have a good sense of humor?
- Do you actively bring humor into your life?
- Do you spend time with people who love to laugh?
- Do you read humorous books and listen to humorous records and tapes?
- Do you have a positive or negative attitude about most things?
- If something unpleasant comes along, are you paralyzed by fear?
- Are you terrified of new opportunities, or do you see them as a new way of applying your skills?
- If your initial attempts at a project do not succeed at first, do you try to create new ways to adjust, or do you quit?
- Do you feel like a victim when things donít go the way that you wish they would?
- Do you see all situations as gifts to be used for gaining new knowledge?
- Are you able to express feelings of joy, love, and sadness?
- Do you hold in your feelings?
- Do you live life with a sense of hopelessness, powerlessness, and frustration?
- Are you patient, tolerant, and compassionate?
- Have you ever taken care of a pet?

## MAKING EXERCISE PART OF YOUR DAILY DIET

If you have been consistent in applying my exercise recommendations throughout the 30-Day Purification Program this is not the time to stop! The exercises that you choose should be the ones that are the most fun and that you feel you will do consistently. With this in mind, it is important to note that there are different physical types. Some physical types will adjust to one athletic activity better than others. After all, the shape of your bones, your coordination, your muscle type, and your reflex speed are all inherited characteristics. Even our body type is basically an inherited characteristic.

Most body types are divided into one of three categories.

1. Muscular persons (mesomorphs) do best in contact sports and court sports.
2. Tall, thin persons (ectomorphs) do best in endurance sports.
3. Obese persons (endomorphs) are less likely to be professional or world-class athletes.

The shape of your body (your morph type) determines the sports that best suit you. With discipline, regularity, and patience you can modify your basic body type.

## CHART

### *Exercise and Body Purification*

Exercise is a key element to maintaining good health and continuing the body purification process after the initial 30 days.

| Activity | Calories Expended/30 min. |
| --- | --- |
| Bicycling (6 mph) | 120 |
| Jogging (5-1/2 mph) | 330 |
| Running (10 mph) | 640 |
| Swimming (25yd/min) | 135 |
| Tennis (singles) | 200 |
| Walking (3mph) | 160 |

Source: Adapted from U.S. Department of Health and Human Services, Exercise and Your Heart (Bethesda, MD: National Institute of Health, 1981).

### HOW TO START EXERCISING

A basic exercise program should include elements of aerobics, stretching, and strengthening exercises. Here is a simple basic program of exercise to start with.

## The Benefits of Aerobics

The easiest way to develop a consistent aerobics program is to commit to 30 minutes of vigorous daily activity at least three times per week. The safest and most popular aerobic exercises include dancing, swimming, vigorous walking, cycling, roller skating, in-line skating, biking, running, race walking, and cross-country skiing.

1. Aerobics burns calories while you exercise and afterwards as well. That's because your metabolism may increase by 10 percent for up to 24 hours following exercise.
2. In addition, with most types of exercise, calories are burned in proportion to body weight: lighterweight people burn fewer calories, heavier people burn more calories.
3. Exercising on a regular basis (for less than an hour) actually helps decrease your appetite.
4. Other benefits from exercise include higher energy levels, better ability to concentrate, and sounder sleep.

## Calories Expended During Various Activities

Aerobic exercise is essential for those attempting to lose weight. The figures in the accompanying chart represent the average calories expended by a 150-pound person. For a 100 pound person, reduce the calories by one-third; for a 200 pound person, multiply by one and one-third.

## STRETCHING

## Myths About Stretching

There is probably no type of exercise that has more myths associated with it than does stretching. It has been the general belief among athletes, for example, that touching the toes, running in place, and otherwise warming up before a workout will prevent muscle injuries. Recent studies, however, indicate this is just not so. Although proper stretching can certainly improve range of motion and make you feel better after a workout, that is the extent of its therapeutic value.

According to Dr. Robert B. Armstrong, a researcher at the

University of Georgia in Athens, "Although warming up and stretching do not protect against muscle injury, it might help prevent the soreness that is sometimes experienced when connective tissue surrounding the muscle fibers has been injured. Stretching would make the connective tissue more elastic and resistant to injury."

### The Five Most Important Rules for Stretching

Clearly it seems that stretching offers great value if done properly, even if it does not ultimately reduce injuries. The key to stretching is to do it properly.

1. Stretch at least three times per week.
2. Avoid overstretching.
3. Remember to stretch if you are involved with heavy, weight-bearing exercises like weight training.
4. Stretching should be done intuitively, moving each joint through its range of motion and feeling the release.
5. Stretching should feel releasing and pleasurable, not painful. It is a simple process and should not be made more complex than is necessary.

NOTE: *The single essential rule for effective stretching is this: Stretch the muscles you have used the most soon after exercising them, and only for as long and as often as it feels good.*

## STRENGTH BUILDING

Strength-building exercises can include certain types of yoga and even aerobic exercise when done with light weights. Most strength-building programs are based on the use of free-standing weights (bar bells, dumb bells) and specialized strength-building machines, such as Universal, Cybex, or Nautilus.

Body building and weight lifting are unique among many exercise approaches in that they require attention to detail, discipline, and a unique sense of self-image.

### Three Benefits of Strength Building

1. Strength building affects primarily the muscles, tendons, and ligaments that are the support system of the body.

2. With strength building joints and cartilage are lubricated and nourished and bones actually thicken.

3. With strength building, there is less chance of injuries and you will have an improved physical appearance.

NOTE: *Unless you are looking specifically to gain bulk or create a sculptured physique, strength training can be easily integrated into a low-impact aerobic program such as the one offered on the following chart:*

| *Activity* | *Comment* |
|---|---|
| *1. Warm-up (5-10 min)* | *Easy activity such as slow walking, cycling, or swimming, followed by stretching.* |
| *2. Aerobics (10-15 min)* | *Low-impact exercise is highly recommended to prevent joint injury. Running and jogging is not recommended in general and especially not for the elderly.* |
| *3. Strength training (15-20 min)* | *Low-intensity muscular endurance training. Activities suggested include calisthenics or hand-crank ergometer. Some individuals who would like a more intense strengthening workout may choose to use free weights and weight-training machines such as Universal, Nautilus, and Cybex machines as part of a strength-building, body-building or power-lifting program.* |
| *4. Cool-down (8-10 min)* | *Mild exercise followed by stretching. Any exercise used in step 1 is adequate.* |
| *5. Meditation (5-30 minutes gradually increasing time)* | *This is not generally included or mentioned in books exercise books and manuals on exercise but is an essential element of fitness nonetheless. Take a few minutes before and after your workouts to thank the divine power for the gift of a functional body (on whatever level it is able to function). When working out, stay focused and be attentive to detail and then let your mind fly into "automatic pilot."* |

## CHARTING THE COURSE

The following chart should help you to clarify which exercises are best for aerobic, stretching, strengthening, or meditation. The chart is based on sports practiced at a recreational, not a professional or highly competitive, level. This is a general chart, and some activities are beneficial in a number of ways and are marked as such. Racquet sports, though vigorous, are not generally aerobic because of the constant stopping between volleys. Some sports like wind sailing, can be aerobic when done competitively, but more often are not aerobic in a recreational form.

| Exercise | Aerobic | Stretching | Strengthening | Meditative |
|---|---|---|---|---|
| Bicycling | • | • | • | • |
| Football | | | • | • |
| Baseball | | | | • |
| Basketball | | | | • |
| Motorbikes | | | | • |
| In-line skating | • | • | • | • |
| Snow skiing | | | • | • |
| Soccer | • | | | • |
| Stickball | | | | • |
| Volleyball | | | | • |
| Ice skating | • | | • | • |
| Sledding | | | | • |
| Gymnastics | | • | • | • |
| Hockey | • | | | • |
| Tennis | | | | • |
| Swimming | • | • | | • |
| Skateboarding | | | | • |
| Racquetball | • | | | • |
| Paddleball | | | | • |
| Squash | • | | | • |
| Bowling | | | | • |
| Horseback riding | | | | • |
| Golf | | | | • |
| Hang gliding | | | | • |

| | | | | |
|---|---|---|---|---|
| *Billiards* | | | | • |
| *Waterskiing* | | | | • |
| *Weight-lifting* | | | • | • |
| *Martial arts* | | • | • | • |
| *Badminton* | | | | • |
| *Cheerleading* | • | • | • | • |
| *Surfing* | | • | | • |
| *Table Tennis* | | • | | • |
| *Trampoline* | • | | | • |
| *Horseshoes* | | | | • |
| *Handball* | | | | • |
| *Cross-country skiing* | • | • | • | • |
| *Mountain climbing* | • | | • | • |
| *Fencing* | | | | • |
| *Stair climbing* | • | | • | • |

# THE WATER CURE: SOOTHE AND BALANCE YOUR BODY USING HYDROTHERAPY

Spas throughout the world use water in one form or another as part of their regular body-purification programs. Soaking tired, aching feet; taking a long, hot shower to wake up in the morning; relaxing in a warm tub at night; or using sauna, steam baths, whirlpools, hot tubs, vaporizers, and humidifiers are all common and easily available forms of hydrotherapy.

People are unique, and so each of us may react differently to hydrotherapy. The particular response will depend on climate, the individual's overall health and vitality level, and other personal factors. If you have any serious medical problems, you should first check with your physician before using hot or cold water therapeutically. For safety's sake, have someone with you during a self-treatment.

## HOT OR COLD WATER?

As a rule, cold water is used for stimulation and to conquer fatigue while warm water is used for relaxation. Hot water is used to relieve various types of aches and pains.

Hydrotherapy is safe if applied properly. Neither very hot nor very cold water should be used when there is a loss of sensation in the skin due to nerve damage or some other condition. In such a situation, hot water can cause serious burns and cold water can cause frostbite, because you will not feel the extremes of temperature. Using extremely hot or cold water excessively can have the same effect; that is, it can cause the nerve damage that leads to desensitization.

## Hot Water for Relaxation

Excessively hot water (above 110 degrees Fahrenheit) loses its therapeutic value and can actually have a negative effect on the body by causing destruction of tissues, congestion of body fluids, desensitizing of nerves, and reducing blood pressure, which can cause dizziness.

Hot water is recommended for sedating the system, relaxing muscle spasms, and relieving pain due to muscle stiffness or irritation. Hot water should not be used

1. When there is swelling or inflammation. The increase of blood flow can cause inflamed, congested blood vessels to rupture.
2. If you are overtired. Heat can cause dizziness by lowering blood pressure.
3. When muscles are flaccid.
4. If you have high or low blood pressure, a heart condition, or diabetes, because of the danger of going into shock.

## Cold Water for Stimulation

Cold water stimulates the system and is effective in reducing swelling, inflammation, and the flow of blood to specific organs or parts. It is also useful for increasing muscle tone. It should not be used

1. When there are open abrasions.
2. In case of diabetes, heart problems, or any condition involving poor circulation.

## BATHS FOR TESION RELEASE

A hot bath should last about fifteen minutes. If the water begins to cool, add more hot water to maintain the temperature. Once you have become conditioned to hot baths, you may want to stay in longer.

Hot baths are valuable for cleansing the skin of bacteria and dead cells, and getting rid of aches and pains caused by muscle strain or diseases such as arthritis, rheumatism and gout. If you are not accustomed to taking hot baths, gradually condition your body by starting with warm water and slowly increasing the temperature.

- Add Epsom salts or Dead Sea salts to the bath water. One or two cups of Epsom salts in a tub of water is extremely good for relieving aches and pains. Although it is sometimes used as a laxative, we recommend it for external use only. Used externally, it stimulates the eliminatory activity of the skin and glands and rids the body of harmful toxins and waste through the pores of the skin. This effect can be obtained with ordinary table salt, but to a lesser extent. Bath salts are available at pharmacies and health food stores.

- After soaking in the tub, rub your body with a loofah (a type of natural-fiber sponge), a natural-bristle bath brush, or a bath mitt.

- Put on a terry-cloth robe after taking a hot bath, get into bed, and cover up well with blankets, particularly your head and feet. You probably will perspire for a while and feel somewhat enervated. Stay in bed for several hours.

- When you get up, dry yourself thoroughly, and gently rub your entire body with a towel dampened with cold water. Then dry again slowly.

- Finish by applying a body-moisturizing oil or lotion.

It is almost miraculous the way a hot bath can help relieve general stiffness and soreness.

## Cold Baths—An Energizing Habit

Cold baths should last only about three or four minutes. They are used primarily to stimulate the circulation of blood, thereby invigorating the entire system. They are also helpful in combatting inflammation and swelling.

On first impact, cold water tightens the superficial capillaries, driving the blood to the inner body. Then the superficial capillaries gradually expand and the blood returns to the surface. The circulation of blood is aroused, and the entire body is energized.

CAUTION: *Because cold water lowers body temperature quickly, do not use for long periods of time.*

### Foot Baths for an Invigorating Feeling

Soaking your feet is a very popular and effective hydrotherapy technique to cleanse the body and relieve tired and aching feet.
Try alternate baths of hot and cold water:

- Fill a tub or basin with enough water so that it is an inch or two above your ankles.
- Start with hot water and soak for three to five minutes.
- Then put your feet in cold water for half a minute to a minute.
- Repeat this sequence three times, ending with cold water.
- When you are finished, dry your feet vigorously.

NOTE: *If you do not feel you can take the alternating hot and cold water, soak your feet in hot water with Epsom salts for about 20 minutes, adding hot water, when necessary, to maintain the temperature. Dry briskly when finished.*

Whichever type of foot bath you use, it is invigorating to finish with a massage to the soles of your feet. Simply rub on a light body oil or cream, and then apply cornstarch. This is guaranteed to leave you feeling refreshed all over.

Another relaxing and energizing hydrotherapy technique for the feet, and the entire body, is to walk barefoot in dewy grass or wet sand for 15 to 30 minutes. Finish by drying and massaging your feet thoroughly and then taking a brisk walk in dry socks and shoes.

HOW HYDROTHERAPY EASED HER MENSTRUAL CRAMPS
AND IMPROVED HER CIRCULATION

*Leslie G. was plagued monthly with aches and pains. Her entire body would feel congested. Hot baths became the solution to her problem. Each day she would take a hot bath for about 15 minutes. As the water began to cool, she would add more hot water to maintain the temperature.*

*She found that the hot baths were valuable not only for reducing her cramping but also for cleansing her skin of bacteria and dead cells. She found that the best way to take a hot bath is to add Epsom salt or Dead Sea salts to the water. One or two cups of Epsom salts seemed to do the trick. A book she had read on hydrotherapy had mentioned that the Epsom salts were useful for stimulating the eliminatory activity of the skin and glands and would help to rid the body of harmful toxins and waste through the pores of the skin.*

*After soaking in the tub Leslie G. rubbed her body with a loofah (a type of natural-fiber sponge), a natural-bristle bath brush, or a bath mitt. It was almost miraculous the way a hot bath could help relieve her menstrual cramps and help improve her circulation.*

## WEEK 5 (DAYS 29 AND 30), DAILY MENU PLANS, EXERCISES, AND MEDITATIONS
### *Menu Plan*

**DAY 29**

Breakfast

*16-oz. Juice Formula #1\**
*1/2 cup nonfat, fruit juice—sweetened granola with a sliced banana*
*8-oz. nonfat yogurt (plain or flavored)*
*Herbal tea or coffee substitute*

Lunch

*6-oz. Pine Nut Tabbouleh\**
*1 cup of a steamed, pleasant-tasting sea vegetable (arame, wakamae, kombu, hijiki, nori)*
*1 medium tomato, sliced*
*1 cup romaine lettuce (choice of Spa Dressing\*)*
*1 medium apple*
Herbal tea or coffee substitute

Dinner

*6-oz. Curry Baked Tempeh\**

---

\* Recipes for starred beverages, main dishes, soups, and sauces may be found in Appendix IV, "Herbs and Spices," Appendix V, "Your Home Guide to Juicing," and Appendix VII, "Purification Recipes."

*1/2 cup steamed green peas*
*2 cups romaine lettuce/alfalfa sprouts with*
*Sweet Dill Dressing\**
*6 oz. baked peaches*
*Herbal tea or coffee substitute*

## Foot Massage

This exercise is great for stopping muscle cramps and relaxing the entire body.

1. Sit on the floor or on a chair.
2. Cross one ankle over the opposite knee.
3. Grasp the sole of your foot in the palm of your hand and moving from heel to toes, firmly squeeze the foot. Knead the foot in the same way that you would knead bread dough.
4. Repeat the same process on the other foot.

*Menu Plan*

### DAY 30

Breakfast
*16 oz. Juice Formula #1*
*1/2 cup nonfat, fruit juice sweetened granola*
*Herbal tea or coffee substitute*

Lunch
*6 oz. Mock Chicken Salad\**
*1 cup mashed potatoes with olive oil and chopped garlic*
*1 medium tomato, sliced*
*2 cups romaine lettuce (choice of Spa Dressing\*)*
*1 medium apple*
*Herbal tea or coffee substitute*

Dinner
*6 oz. Spicy Mushroom-Sage Stuffing\**
*1 cup of a steamed, pleasant-tasting sea vegetable (arame, wakamae, kombu, hijiki, nori)*
*2 cups romaine lettuce*

> *6 oz. of any cooked vegetables with Sweet
> and Sour Sauce\* or Chinese Hot Sauce\**
> *8 oz. nonfat yogurt (plain or flavored)*
> *Choices of beverage*

## The Yoga Cobra

The purpose of this exercise is not only to increase flexibility, but also to strengthen the internal organs, increase circulation, and strengthen the gluteal and chest muscles.

1. Lie on your stomach.
2. Bend your elbows and place your hands at the sides of your chest.
3. Raise your chest and feet at the same time holding this position initially for the count of five.
4. Slowly lower your body.
5. Repeat three times.
6. To increase the level of difficulty, hold the position for the count of 10 and repeat 5 to 10 times.

## SUGGESTED GROCERY LIST FOR WEEK 5 (DAYS 29 AND 30)

*Vegetables*: Medium tomato, romaine lettuce (or boston in selected recipes), green peas, alfalfa sprouts, white potatoes, fresh mushrooms, celery, carrots, scallions, beet, cucumber

*Fresh Fruit*: Apple, peaches, lemon or lime, banana

*Spices (dried)*: Onion powder, paprika, curry powder, cayenne pepper powder

Nonfat, fruit juice-sweetened granola

Herbal tea or coffee substitute

Non-fat yogurt (plain or flavored)

Unroasted pine nuts

Bulghur (cracked wheat)

*Fresh Herbs*: Parsley, fresh mint leaves, fresh dill, fresh garlic

Honey

Apple cider vinegar

Raisins or dried currants
Almond oil or extra virgin olive oil
White of black peppercorns
Tempeh
Low-fat yogurt
Roasted almonds
Dijon mustard
TVP (textured vegetable protein)
Eggless tofu-based mayonnaise
Slivered almonds
Distilled water

# NINETEEN BEANS AND SEEDS TO HELP YOU DETOXIFY AND REJUVENATE YOUR BODY

## I

Beans, nuts, and seeds are among the most versatile foods available. They are rich in fiber, natural oils, and protein and are inexpensive and easy to prepare. Because they lack some of the key essential amino acids, combine these foods with a grain whenever possible.

Have your beans with whole grain bread, pasta, or add some whole grain berries to increase the "protein power" of your meal.

### ADUKI BEANS

These are small, maroon-colored beans that are popular in the Far East. They are related to the larger red beans, pinto beans, and red kidney beans but have a distinct, less "beany" taste. Kidney beans are red and shaped like a kidney. They lend themselves to Mexican dishes, especially chili. Aduki beans are great served with rice, or they can be mashed and used as a substitute for tomato paste on pizza or in casseroles. The hard, uncooked aduki bean can be ground into a meal and added to baked goods. **NUTRITION**: Aduki beans have some vitamins and a good amount of phosphorus, calcium, iron, and protein.

## ALMONDS

Almonds are fruits of sweet almond trees, which are related to roses and peaches. The nuts are sold in the shell or shelled, raw or roasted, whole or sliced, slivered, chopped, blanched (skins removed), and flavored. In general, the more processing involved, the more they will cost. One pound of almonds in the shell equals 1 to 1 1/2 cups of shelled nuts. Besides using almonds for baked goods or shakes, you can add them to casseroles, vegetable dishes, and salads. Almond butter is available in health food stores and is a fine alternative to peanut butter. **NUTRITION**: Almonds are high in protein and unsaturated fat, and they contain potassium, phosphorus, calcium, iron and B-vitamins.

## BLACK BEANS

Also called "turtle" beans, these beans are of medium size and slightly square shape. They have a hearty and robust flavor and are popular in Mexico and southwestern United States. Select these beans for thick soups. They are often used in Mediterranean and South American dishes. **PREPARATION**: A traditional way to use black beans is to cook them for soup. They are great as refried beans and can be added to salads and casseroles. When mashed with spices and bread crumbs, they make a wonderful "black bean cake." To cook, soak overnight in four times as much water as beans, and heat for 1-1/2 hour or until tender. In a pressure cooker, use water to cover the beans and cook for about 20 minutes at full pressure.
**NUTRITION**: Black beans contain high amounts of potassium, magnesium, and phosphorus. They also contain smaller amounts of vitamins A, $B_1$, $B_2$, and niacin. Black beans are also a good source of calcium and protein.

## BLACK-EYED PEAS

Black-eyed peas are white, medium-sized seeds with a black eye, or center. They are popular in the southern United States and in Latin American countries. Other names for them are cowpeas, black-eyed beans, and china beans. They are served as a main dish vegetable and are popular in southern and soul food cookery. **PREPARATION:** Black-eyed peas are a "soft" bean and need no soaking prior to cooking. They require only about an hour of cooking or cook with a pressure cooker for about 15 minutes using just enough water to cover the peas. Try black-eyed peas and greens for a Southern-styled dish, or add to soups, salads, and casseroles. **NUTRITION:** Black-eyed peas are a good source of vitamin A, magnesium, and potassium, and they contain B-vitamins, vitamin C, calcium, phosphorus, iron, and protein.

## CHICK PEAS (GARBANZOS)

Chickpeas are one of the more interesting looking beans, being of different color and shape than most other beans. Also called garbanzo beans, they have been a staple food in the Middle East for centuries. These beans are characterized by a nutlike flavor that lends itself to pureeing for dips and main dishes. Seasoned with salt and pepper, the cooked beans are often served cold for snacking. **PREPARATION:** Because chickpeas are quite hard, they need to be soaked before cooking. Add four times as much water as you have beans and cook for three hours. With a pressure cooker, just cover the soaked beans with water and cook for 15 minutes at full pressure. Cooked chickpeas are often eaten with tahini (sesame paste). Lemon juice and seasonings can be added to make hummus and, when cooked, falafel. Their nutty flavor makes chickpeas good for salads, soups, and casseroles. When I was a child, I remember going to weddings or to other family affairs where cooked, cold chickpeas were served. They seemed like a nut to me but tasted different and had a softer texture. Chickpeas are tasty as a roasted snack, or they can be sprouted like other beans. **NUTRITION:** Chickpeas contain high amounts of calcium, phosphorus, potassium, and protein, with notable quantities of iron, zinc, vitamin A, and some B-vitamins.

## FLAX SEEDS

Flaxseeds have become increasingly popular in recent years. Flaxseed oil, which must be refrigerated, is especially rich in Omega-3, an essential fatty acid, that has been shown to slow down the body's ability to make cholesterol. Flaxseeds aid digestion, especially of heavy-fiber foods such as whole grains. They are also a mild laxative. **NUTRITION:** Flaxseeds are high in protein and are rich in many other essential nutrients especially the Omega-3 fatty acid. **PREPARATION:** Flaxseeds can be used in a variety of ways. Substitute flaxseeds for 1/16 of the flour in bread, muffin, or other pastry recipes. Add some to rice dishes and breakfast cereals or sprinkle some on your salad.

## GREAT NORTHERN BEANS

Great northern beans are white beans quite similar to the smaller but more popular navy beans. Most great northerns are grown in western United States. Use these beans for soups, casseroles, or sandwich spreads. **NUTRITION:** Great northerns are a good source of protein, They also contain minerals and B-vitamins.

## LENTILS

Lentils are one of the oldest foods known to humans. They were found buried in pottery jars of ancient Troy and in Bronze Age ruins in Switzerland. These disc-shaped seeds are green, yellow, or brown in color, flat, and about the size of a pea. These cook in only 30 to 45 minutes and do not need soaking. Any extra liquid makes excellent soup or gravy. Lentils team up well with other vegetables, grains, meat, or fruit. **PREPARATION:** Lentils might have been the first "convenience" food, because they are quick and easy to prepare. They need no soaking and only 30 to 60 minutes cooking time. With a pressure cooker it takes about 10 minutes at full pressure; reduce the amount of water so as to cover the lentils in the cooker. Lentils are great for soups, stews, and gravies, blending well with most vegetables. Lentils can also be sprouted as you would other seeds. **NUTRITION:** The minerals phosphorous, potassium, and iron are present in lentils, as are vitamin A, B-vitamins, zinc, copper, and protein.

## LIMA BEANS

These are cream-colored beans with fine ridges coming out from the center. Sometimes called "butter beans," limas are used almost exclusively in North and South America, being unknown in most other parts of the world. Two types are sold: the large "potato lima" and the small "baby." **NUTRITION:** Limas are high in protein, iron, potassium, and phosphorus and contain B-vitamins.

## MUNG BEANS

Mung beans are small green beans that are used extensively in East Asian countries and are gaining popularity in North America. **PREPARATION:** Although they can be cooked as you would other beans, mung beans are usually sprouted. Just soak overnight, using 2 tablespoons mung beans per cup of water. Drain off the water in the morning and put beans in a quart-size jar, then cover with a screen or cheesecloth. Put in a dark cupboard at a slight angle and remember to rinse the beans two or three times a day for three to five days. After sprouting, refrigerate until ready to use. They can be added to salads, sandwiches, and oriental dishes. **NUTRITION:** Raw mung bean sprouts are high in vitamins A and C and potassium, as well as containing B-vitamins, phosphorus, calcium, and iron. **STORAGE:** Sprouts should be used in ten days.

## PEANUTS

The pods grow underground like potatoes and are harvested similarly. Raw peanuts are sold in the shell or shelled (usually Spanish or Valencia types), and many are available roasted and salted in the shell or as cocktail nuts. **PREPARATION:** You can cook peanuts as you would beans; soak raw nuts overnight; then cover with water and simmer for 2 hours. Raw or roasted peanuts can be added to casseroles, soups, and baked goods. **NUTRITION:** Peanuts are high in protein. They are about 50 percent oil, most of this being unsaturated, and are good sources of niacin and thiamine.

## PEAS

Peas are the seeds of certain legumes that have been a staple food for centuries. They are sold in various forms:

- Whole green peas, which have been dried and shelled from the pod
- Green split peas, which have the outer seed coat removed and are divided into two halves

- Whole yellow and yellow split peas, which are of a different variety, color, and taste (milder) than green peas

**PREPARATION:** Since they cook in a relatively short period of time and do not require soaking, peas can be cooked along with rice or other grains for a rich protein dish. Dried peas are good for soups, casseroles and salads. Split peas need no soaking. Use 2 to 3 parts fresh water to 1 part peas, boil 30 to 60 minutes, and cool. Pressure cooking takes 5 to 10 minutes at full pressure. **NUTRITION:** Peas are excellent sources of protein, vitamin A, iron and contain some B-vitamins.

## SESAME SEEDS

Sesame seeds are small, light-brown seeds from the sesame plant. They are often found on breads and buns, but are increasingly being used as a nutritious addition to other foods. **PREPARATION:** Add sesame seeds to soups, salads, cereals, or cooked vegetables. Grind them with salt to make gomasio, a tasty seasoning, or toast and grind them into a meal and add to baked goods. Mixed with peanuts or chickpeas, sesame seeds are a protein-rich food. **NUTRITION:** Besides protein, sesame seed are high in an oil that is rich in vitamin E. They are one of the best sources of calcium and also contain iron, phosphorus, potassium, and B-vitamins.

## SOYBEANS

Of all the beans and legumes none are as protein rich as the soybean. Before the 1960s most Americans had never heard of soybeans, unless of course they read farming magazines, since these beans were used primarily to feed cattle. And yet at the same time soybeans were being used in the Orient in over four hundred different ways. Chinese literature over three thousand years old makes mention of soybeans.

To the uninitiated, soybean based foods, commonly called soy-foods, can seem exotic and confusing. In fact they are easy to use and highly nutritious as well as easily available in many forms. Unlike many other beans which lack certain essential amino acids, the protein content of soybeans is almost equal to that of meat and eggs. Soybeans are also a good source of fiber, high-quality oil, lecithin (a fat emulsifier), and many other nutrients. When buying and using soyfoods, it is important to know how to read the labels. As in all manufactured foods there are higher-quality and lower-quality products. The more information you have the more intelligent your purchasing decisions will be. **PREPARATION, NUTRITION, AND STORAGE:** Soybeans are not generally served the same way that other beans are served as in a soup or as a side dish. Instead they are eaten in various processed forms such as soy milk or tofu. The nutritional values and storage directions will be different for these foods. (See the soyfoods discussion later in this appendix.)

## SUNFLOWER SEEDS

Sunflower seeds are from flowers in the daisy family. They grow inside the flower head surrounded by bright yellow petals. The black, striped shells contain the nutritious kernels. You can buy them raw in the shell or hulled, or roasted and salted. **PREPARATION:** Substitute sunflower seed kernels for nuts in any recipe. They are great with brown rice or mixed in bean casseroles. Grind sunflower seeds into a meal and mix them with peanut butter for a tasty spread. You can also sprout sunflower seeds as you would other seeds. **NUTRITION:** They are high in protein and unsaturated fat, and contain calcium, phosphorus, iron, B-vitamins, and vitamins A and D. Sprouts have vitamin C.

# EIGHT SIMPLE STEPS FOR COOKING BEANS

1. Always cook the beans in the water they were soaked in. If the beans begin to stick to the pot, add more water. Keep the heat low. When you cook beans on a high flame, they will begin to break up, become mushy, and stick to the pot.

2. Don't overcook the beans if you plan to reheat them later. For bean dishes that require reheating, as well as for beans that will be refrigerated or used in salads, the beans should be tender but still hold their shape. Cook the beans until they are very soft if you intend to puree or mash them. Split peas and lentils will be tender in about 45 minutes. Most other beans require 2 to 3 hours.

3. If you are preparing a recipe using beans, add the salt or other spices when the other ingredients are added to the beans. Salt hardens most beans and increases the cooking time.

4. Some cookbooks recommend adding baking soda to the water. This decreases cooking time and makes the skins separate from the beans easily. Unfortunately, baking soda also destroys the B-vitamin thiamine. Never add baking soda to dried beans.

5. Remember that beans expand when they cook. One cup of dry beans (approximately 1/2 pound) will yield 2 to 3 cups after cooking. Be sure that you use a pot large enough to accommodate this expansion.

6. Rinse the beans in cold water.

7. Dried beans and whole peas should be soaked before cooking to replace water lost in drying and to reduce cooking time. Lentils and split peas are the exception to this rule. Most beans should be soaked in three times their volume of water overnight. The few that require four times their volume are noted. A quick method of preparation is to bring the beans and water to a boil and then cook them for 2 minutes. Then remove the beans from the heat, cover them, and let them soak for 2 hours. I always use distilled water for soaking and cooking my beans.

8. When you have finished soaking them, bring the beans and water to a boil, reduce to a very low heat, cover, and simmer gently until they are tender. This should take about 2 hours.

## THE SIMPLE WAY TO BUY BEANS

Most dried legumes are available in see-through packages or in bulk.

- Look for a package with beans of uniform size. Small beans cook faster than large ones, and a variety of sizes will result in uneven cooking, causing large beans to be soft while the small ones will break up and become mushy.

- Check for color. Dried beans should have a bright, uniform color. Fading color is an indication that the bean has been in storage too long. Older beans take longer to cook and can be tasteless.

- Look for bags of beans that are free of any visible defects. These can include discolorations, cracked coating, foreign materials, and perforations and tears in the package itself.

# STORING BEANS FOR LONG-TERM FRESHNESS

All dry edible legumes are best stored in closed containers in a cool, airtight, dry place or refrigerated. This will maintain the nutritional quality of the food and also reduce pest infestation.

# SOYFOODS

In the last 30 years soybeans and soybean-based products (soyfoods) have exploded onto the American marketplace. This expanding popularity of soyfoods has come largely through the increase of interest in vegetarianism, macrobiotics, and oriental cooking styles. Among the soyfoods most commonly available are

Soy nuts
Grits
Flour
Protein powder
Oil
Tempeh
Tofu
Soy sauce
Miso
Lecithin
Meat substitutes
TVP (textured vegetable protein)
Dairy-free imitation "soy" ice cream.

Vegetarians are often looking for new protein substitutes especially those that can mimic the texture and taste of animal foods such as eggs, chicken, beef, or meat. Macrobiotics, a specialized system of diet and life-style for building and maintaining optimal health, uses large amounts of soyfoods, especially miso, soy sauce, and tofu.

### TOFU: THE VERSATILE PROTEIN

Tofu, a custard like food made from soybeans, is the most popular and versatile of all the soyfoods. A complete protein containing all eight essential amino acids, tofu is very low in saturated fat and has no cholesterol. Over 1-billion people use this food as their primary source of daily protein. Tofu has been the foundation of the oriental diet for several thousand years.

As more and more Americans recognized the health benefits of tofu, the natural foods industry began integrating it into pizzas, custards, taco fillings, desserts, and so on. Because of its versatility, tofu is gaining increasing popularity as a high-quality vegetable protein source.

Tofu comes in three textures: soft, firm, and extra-firm. The extra-firm tofu can be dehydrated, shaped in the form of noodles, or dried and shredded. Mixed with other ingredients, tofu can be prepared to look like hot dogs, sausage, or cream cheese. In its basic form, tofu is generally sold either loose or in plastic, sealed, water-filled tubs.

### The Benefits of Adding Tofu to Most of Your Meals?

1. Tofu is an excellent source of protein, containing all eight essential amino acids.
2. Tofu is low in saturated fats, calories, and sodium.
3. Tofu contains no cholesterol.
4. Tofu is an excellent replacement for foods such as eggs, milk, cheese, and meat.
5. Tofu can be used creatively in cooking to make stuffed tamales, tofu pizza, and so on.

## SOY SAUCE

Soy sauce (shoyu) is a black, brewed, salty liquid that has been widely used as a seasoning in Oriental cuisine and in macrobiotic cooking. It is now popular for all types of food and is found even in the most traditional American kitchens. Soy sauce is an excellent condiment with a variety of uses in cooking. Tamari is a type of soy sauce that, though similar in appearance and flavor to common soy sauce, has a stronger, sharper flavor and aroma. Tamari is brewed from soybeans and sea salt, while common soy sauce often is brewed with wheat to produce a mellower flavor.

The name Tamari applies to a liquid that is a natural by-product of miso (fermented soy beans). Many commercial Tamari products, even many so-called "natural" brands, commonly use cheap ingredients and chemical additives to make a profitable product. One popular trick is to use cheap, nutritionally inferior defatted soybeans rather than whole ones. The fermentation time is reduced from 15 months to less than half that time through use of hydrochloric acid, monosodium glutamate, and waste water. Caramel coloring is commonly used to mask poor color, and alcohol or sodium benzoate may be added as a preservative. Many other such tricks have been devised by the soy sauce industry, yet none of them is used by high-quality soy sauce manufacturers. A superior soy sauce should have a rich, full-bodied flavor and aroma and a pleasant, fragrant bouquet, full of subtle textures. It will have a range of tastes that continue to stimulate your palate and improve the flavor of your food. Inferior soy sauce will have a sharp, pungent smell, with a salty, narrow taste. It may even have a slightly "chemical" or "artificial" smell. High-quality Tamari is a much superior product and is consistently and carefully brewed from whole soybeans, pure well water, and mineral-rich sea salt. It is aged naturally for a minimum of two years.

When choosing soy sauce, pick a brand that is free of preservatives. Reduced-salt varieties are also desirable. Beware of any brands that contain preservatives, especially sodium benzoate.

## MISO: BLACK GOLD

This thick black paste is a traditional Japanese seasoning, generally made from soybeans, though other grains and beans may be used in its preparation.

High-quality, authentic miso is crafted by naturally fermenting whole soybeans and whole cereal grains. The best miso is naturally crafted and fermented for one to two years by very old traditional techniques, often by a small, family shop using inherited techniques.

Cheaper, commercial miso and some so-called "natural" brands are mass produced. They are commonly made from cheap, defatted soybeans that have had their nutritious oil removed by a high-heat, solvent process. Producers of these types of miso commonly use surplus grains stored several years fermented with cheap soybean meal. To compensate for poor ingredients, such producers commonly use flavor enhancers and other chemicals, artificial colorings, preservatives, and sweeteners. Much of the value of miso is based on the fermenting bacteria in it. One of the principal benefits of miso are the beneficial microorganisms that cause the miso to ferment, and also aid human digestion. These microorganisms are destroyed during pasteurization. Most miso sold in America, including so-called "natural" brands, are neither made from organically grown ingredients, nor are they unpasteurized. In fact most of these misos are commonly pasteurized by either irradiation or a high-temperature process in order to increase the shelf life of the product. Unfortunately, this destroys the microorganisms as well.

Remember that the best miso, like soy sauce, is made with whole organically grown soybeans, water, and sea salt. It should be a product that is free of synthetic ingredients and should be unpasteurized. Unpasteurized miso should be refrigerated. Miso is moist and for this reason it may mold if not refrigerated or stored in a cool place. The mold is not harmful and may be scraped off or mixed into the miso. Miso is wonderful in soups, mixed with tahini (sesame butter), as a spread for bread, and as a general seasoning.

## TEMPEH: A GREAT MEAT SUBSTITUTE

Tempeh is another fermented soy product, but unlike miso and soy sauce, which are used as seasonings, tempeh is used as a food. Used by over 100 million Indonesians as their staple food, the making of tempeh uses over half the entire annual Indonesian soybean crop. In its native land, Tempeh is generally sold as 4-cubic-inch "cylinders" wrapped in banana leaves. In the United States, tempeh is sold as an 8-oz., flat, rectangular patty. Tempeh is made by soaking, dehulling, and boiling soybeans. These beans are then mixed with a starter culture ( a piece of tempeh from a previous batch), much the way that that a new batch of yogurt can be made by adding live yogurt culture to milk.

Tempeh is even more nutritionally balanced than tofu since it has live cultures and because, unlike tofu, tempeh can be made from soybeans mixed with other cereal grains, such as millet, barley, or rice, thus increasing its value as a source of complete protein. Fresh tempeh has the aroma of fresh baked bread and a rich, earthy taste—sort of a cross between nuts and mushrooms.

Tempeh can be used as a meat substitute and can be baked, steamed, boiled, or stir fried. Tempeh is less versatile than tofu since tempeh has a strong distinctive taste and thus cannot be blended into other foods as easily as tofu. It is available in various forms at your local natural foods store.

## OTHER SOY FOODS

*Lecithin:* A natural emulsifier that is used in some diets in the belief that it may assist in the breakdown of fatty tissue. It is also an excellent source of the nutrients choline and inositol.

*Soy Flour:* Very finely ground soybeans. Soy flour is often added to whole grain flour to increase the protein content of bread.

*Soy Grits:* These are coarsely ground soybeans. They are used in making stews and other vegetarian dishes.

*Soy Nuts:* These are not nuts at all but rather soybeans that have been roasted in oil and salted. They are high in calories and fat and are somewhat similar in taste and texture to dry roasted peanuts. I do not recommend them due to the high rancidity factor and fat content.

*Soy Margarine:* This is simply artificially hydrogenated soy oil with beta carotene added to make it yellow like butter. This highly saturated fat is usually high in sodium as well and should be avoided.

*Soy Protein Powder:* This is often used as a base for powdered nutritional supplements or as a substitute for egg and milk protein.

*Soy Oil:* Good for cooking and in salads.

*Meat and Dairy Substitutes*: Soybeans are so versatile that manufacturers have used them as fillers with meat or pork in the making of sausage. McDonald's has even started making a soy burger for its restaurants in Holland. Many health food companies have found that by combining soybeans and soybean derivatives they can create substitutes for many foods, including hot dogs, cream cheese, chicken salad, egg salad, margarine, and ice cream. TVP (textured vegetable protein) can be made to have the texture of sausage, chicken or ground beef and when mixed with oil, spices, and other ingredients can be used to produce a highly nutritious and flavorful substitute.

# GRAINS:
# AN EXPLOSION
# OF GOOD
# NUTRITION

## II

Within each whole grain berry or kernel, nature has packed all the elements necessary to reproduce life. So long as it remains intact in this form, it will keep indefinitely.

When the pharaohs of ancient Egypt died, they were buried with all the material they would need to sustain them in their journey into the great unknown. In uncovering some of these tombs, scientists have found large earthenware jars full of wheat that they have been able to sprout, even though it was over four thousand years old.

A whole grain consists of the bran, germ, and endosperm. Most grain based foods that we are most familiar with are refined, that is, they have been stripped of the bran, and often of the germ as well.

## BRAN

In the last few years we have heard a lot about the value of bran.

First, wheat bran was publicized as a source of fiber that could help reduce colon cancer. Then, the media publicized some preliminary and controversial studies that indicated that oat bran could reduce cholesterol levels. The public spent millions of dollars on high-bran cereals without even knowing what bran was. Most of these products were highly processed and refined with bran added back in. When taken as part of a whole grain, bran is a valuable source of nutrition. This outermost part of the grain is a source of fiber as well as B-vitamins, proteins, fats, and minerals. Raw, unprocessed bran is recognized for its ability to promote the speedy movement of food wastes through the bowel, as well as helping to maintain stable blood sugar levels. Some bran is better than no bran, but a whole grain cereal with the bran intact is the best choice.

### WHEAT GERM, WHEAT GERM OIL

Wheat germ and wheat germ oil are rich sources of vitamins E, B, and A, protein, and essential unsaturated fatty acids.

### THE ENDOSPERM

This is the part of the grain most familiar to Americans, because it is what remains after the bran and the germ have been processed out after the milling. It is a source of complex carbohydrates and virtually nothing else of importance to health. Most of us see the endosperm in the form of unbleached white flour.

Whole grains are rich in fiber, vitamins, minerals, and protein.

## THIRTEEN WHOLE GRAINS TO DETOXIFY AND REGENERATE YOUR BODY

### AMARANTH

This grain, slightly larger than millet, was the primary grain used by the ancient Aztecs of South America. It is rich in high-quality protein, second only to to quinoa. Amaranth is high in the amino acid lysine, which is not present in most grains. While it can be cooked into a hot cereal, it is most often added to other whole grain cereals to improve their protein balance.

## BARLEY

A delicious chewy grain similar to wheat, barley is one of the main ingredients in beer. *Hulled* barley is the whole berry with only the inedible outer layers removed. *Pearled* barley is grain with all of the husks processed off. *Malted* barley has been sprouted and then toasted. **PREPARATION:** Hulled barley takes 1 1/2 hours to cook and uses 2 1/2 to 3 cups of water. Pealed barley takes 25 to 30 minutes to cook, using 2 cups water to 1 cup grain. Malted barley flour is great for malted milk shakes. The cooked grain can be used in soups and casseroles or as a side dish. Rolled barley and barley flakes take 10 to 20 minutes to cook depending on the size of the flakes (use 2 to 3 parts water to 1 part oats). **NUTRITION:** Hulled barley contains protein, niacin, thiamine, and most minerals. *Pearling* reduces the fiber and protein considerably. **STORAGE:** Put barley in an airtight and bugproof container in a dry, cool place.

## BUCKWHEAT GROATS

You wouldn't know it to look at it but the buckwheat "grain" is actually a fruit. The name was derived from bockweit, a Dutch term meaning "beechwheat," because of its resemblance to beechnuts and nutritional similarities to wheat. Buckwheat seeds are called groats; coarse-ground groats are grits. Groats have a strong and robust flavor, and are typically used to make pancakes and pasta. Buckwheat without the hull is available roasted and unroasted, with the former called kasha.

Buckwheat pancake mix is flour with a leavening agent and other dry ingredients. **PREPARATION:** Buckwheat groats can be cooked into a breakfast cereal, as can grits. Saute grain until toasted. Add 2 to 2 1/2 times amount of boiling water. Cover and simmer 10 to 20 minutes. The groats may also be toasted and eaten as a snack or made for pancakes and dumplings. **NUTRITION:** Rich in vitamin E, calcium and the B-complex vitamins, phosphorus, and protein. **STORAGE:** Buckwheat is best stored in a cool, dry place. Keep flours refrigerated.

## BULGAR

Bulgar, a form of processed wheat, is quick to prepare and nutritious to eat. It has an appealing nutty flavor and is made by boiling wheat kernels, drying them, removing some of the bran layers, and finally cracking the kernels. **PREPARATION:** Bulgar can be mixed with fruits, salads, vegetables, meats, poultry, and fish or eaten by itself. You can boil, bake, fry, or roast it, or just soak in water for a few hours, since it is already precooked. To recook it, heat a small amount of oil in a deep pan and saute the grain until all bits are coated. Add 1 1/2 times its amount of boiling water or stock. Cover and simmer about 10 minutes. In bread recipes, use about 1 cup bulgur to 5 cups flour. **NUTRITION:** Bulgar has the same nutrients as whole wheat but in smaller quantities. It is rich in protein and in riboflavin, niacin, and thiamine. **STORAGE:** Bulgar may be stored for longer periods than most grain because it is precooked and dried. Keep it in a cool, dry place free from insects.

## CORN

The only grain containing beta-carotene, corn is probably the most versatile of all grains. It can be milled into flakes, grits, and meal, but this involves removing the bran and germ and thus the corn's nutrients. There are various types of corn including blue, yellow, and white. Yellow corn has more vitamin A than white corn. Another corn variety is "flint" or "dent" corn. Also called field corn, dent corn is the basis for hot cereals like cornmeal or mush, tortilla and polenta. Corn meal or flour is ground from "dent" corn. Grits are usually small pieces of white corn, and hominy is the inside starchy part of the kernel. Corn pancake mix is corn flour with a leaving agent and other dry ingredients mixed in. Blue corn has more protein, iron, manganese, and potassium than any other variety. There is also a high-lysine corn, developed with up to 70 percent more lysine than ordinary corn. Corn can be combined with legumes to provide a complete meal protein. In many parts of our own country, primarily in the South, whole corn and products made from corn have been basic in the people's diet for many generations. If you look on any package of commercially prepared corn meal in your market, you will note the words "degermed." This means that the germ of life has been removed to gain extended shelf life.

From this corn germ, we get corn oil, and we consume the corn meal, which, in reality, is just the dead residue containing primarily starch.

**PREPARATION:** Eat fresh corn raw, steamed, or baked. Corn meal is great for muffins and cornbread, and the flour is used in tortillas or as a breading. Grits and hominy are cooked as cereal dishes. **NUTRITION:** In addition to beta-carotene corn has plus B-vitamins, protein, and minerals. **STORAGE:** Store in covered containers, and refrigerate ground products for freshness.

## COUSCOUS

Couscous is made from coarsely ground durum wheat (semolina) that has been precooked. It is a light grain that can be recooked in just 5 to 10 minutes. **PREPARATION:** Bring 1 1/4 cups water or broth to boil. Add 2 tablespoons canola oil, 1 cup couscous, and salt if desired. (For whole wheat couscous, use 1 1/2 cups water to 1 cup couscous.) Stir and cover. Remove from heat and allow to stand for 5 minutes. Stir to fluff; serve (makes 2—3 servings). Serve with vegetables and seasonings as a main or side dish for dinner; as a tasty breakfast cereal with milk, honey, and raisins; as a salad or dessert. **STORAGE:** Store in a closed container in a cool, dry place.

## MILLET

Millet is one of the oldest foods known to humans. It is a highly nutritious grain. Millet is cultivated mostly in regions with primitive agricultural practices. In the United States millet is produced mostly for birdseed or cattle grain. This grain has high-quality protein, significant iron content, and a good balance of essential amino acids. It can be eaten by itself as a whole grain hot cereal, mixed with other grains in cold cereals or puffed. It is generally well tolerated by people with wheat allergies. **PREPARATION:** Millet is cooked with 2 parts water or stock to 1 part grain in about 30 minutes. Presoaking adds a wonderful flavor and texture. Cooked or leftover millet is good in casseroles, breads, or for a breakfast cereal. Millet flour can be made by grinding millet seeds in a regular food mill. The flour is a great addition to breads, pie crusts, and crackers. Sprouted millet is also good for cereals. **NUTRITION:** Millet is high in B-complex vitamins (more so than most grains) and is rich in protein with many of the essential amino acids present. It is very high in potassium and low in sodium. **STORAGE:** Kept dry and away from pests, millet can be stored for two years.

## OATS

Oats are one of the most popular of all the grains. It is commonly eaten as hot cereal, cold cereal, and as pure oat bran. Though oat bran has more concentrated fiber content, it is refined. It is best to use whole oats since all forms of oats contain soluble fiber. Oats are high in protein, sodium, and unsaturated fat. This versatile grain can be made into cereal, added to bread and cookies, and even made into creamlike base for soups. Old-fashioned oats cook in 5 minutes. **PREPARATION:** Boil 3/4 cups of water in a covered saucepan; stir in 1/3 cup of oats. oats. Return to a boil; reduce heat, continuing to boil. Cook uncovered about 5 minutes, stirring occasionally. Remove from heat. (Optional) Cover and let stand until it achieves the desired thickness. For creamier oatmeal, combine water, salt, and oats, bring to a boil. Cook as directed.

## QUINOA

First cultivated by the Incas, quinoa is a "supergrain" with complete protein and more protein than any other grain. It is a good source of starch, sugars, oil, fiber, minerals, vitamin F, and B-complex vitamins. It is versatile as a hot cereal or combined with other grains in ready-to-eat cereal. Quinoa flour is used in pastries and can be made into pasta.

## RICE

A staple food for more than half of the world's people, rice comes in long-, medium-, and short-grain varieties. Brown rice is rice with its indigestible husk removed, but is still the whole kernel and is rich in nutrients such as the B-vitamins, iron, vitamin F, amino acids, and linoleic acid. On the other hand, white rice has the husk plus several other outer layers and germ removed, and is much less nutritious. In unprocessed brown rice, nature has put most of the goodness in the outer coating. When we remove this outer coating, we have white rice, which is primarily "empty calories." The best nutrients went with the husks.

Brown rice is used in natural foods cereals, ground to form rice cream as a hot cereal and can be puffed. White rice has the husk plus several other outer layers and germ removed, and is much less nutritious than the brown variety. White rice is the variety used in refined, processed cereals.

Brown rice is used in natural foods cereals, ground to form rice cream as a hot cereal and puffed. To ensure full flavor and nutrition, nothing is removed but the husk. Short-grain brown rice tends to be moist and chewy. Long grain brown rice is drier and fluffier when cooked. Sweet brown rice is moist and sweet—well suited for puddings. Suggestion: Cook a week's supply of brown rice and store in a covered container in the refrigerator or freezer. If rice becomes compacted, rinse in cold water before reheating.

One of the most tasty of the rices is Basmati rice. Basmati rice smells like buttered peanuts and has a memorable nutty flavor and fluffy texture. The cooked grain almost doubles in length yet changes little in thickness. This prized rice variety originated in the foothills of the Himalayas. Brown basmati is a whole grain rice, while white basmati has had its outer layers removed by polishing. **NUTRITION:** Whole grain basmati is low in fat and a good source of fiber, minerals, and the B-complex vitamins. White basmati has lost some of its nutrients during the polishing process. **PREPARATION:** Rinse rice thoroughly and place one part rice to 2 parts water in a saucepan. Bring to a vigorous boil; lower heat. When water is just bubbling, cover the pot, continuing to simmer. Cook whole grain basmati for 45 minutes and white basmati for 20—25 minutes. Do not remove lid during cooking. Remove from heat, allow to steam, still covered, for 10 to 15 minutes. Fluff rice with fork before serving. **STORAGE:** Store in a closed container in a cool, dry place.

## RYE

Rye is a cereal grass second only to wheat for breads. Rye berries are the whole grain. Dark or whole rye flour contains most of the berry which has been ground. Light rye flour has had some of the bran removed. Rye meal and rye cereal are coarse ground berries, and rolled rye is steamed and pressed flat like rolled oats. **PREPARATION:** Cook berries using 2 parts water to 1 part grain and cook for 1 to 2 hours. They're good cooked with rice 2 to 1 (rice to rye). Rye flour and meal can be added to breads and other baked goods, and rye cereal is good to cook for breakfast, using about 2 1/2 cups of water to 1 cup cereal and cooked for 30 minutes. Rolled rye can be used as you would rolled oats. **NUTRITION:** Quite similar to wheat, rye contains B-vitamins, vitamin E, protein, iron, and several minerals. **STORAGE:** Store rye in a cool, dry place away from pests. Whole rye stores up to three years; ground products should be refrigerated and used frequently to maintain freshness.

## WHEAT

Wheat is by far the most popular grain in this country. Americans eat about 115 pounds each year, mostly as bread. This grain comes in many varieties. Hard wheat contains higher levels of protein, while soft wheat has more carbohydrates. Wheat that has been broken into small pieces by coarse milling is called cracked wheat, while another type of wheat, durum, is used exclusively for pasta. Semolina is refined durum flour, couscous is made of either durum wheat or millet, and bulgur is cracked wheat that has been partially cooked and toasted. Couscous is a hot wheat cereal made of either durum wheat or millet. Although it is generally refined, it can be made as well from whole grains. Wheatena is a ground wheat cereal that is served hot. **PREPARATION:** Wheat berries, are good for casseroles, soups or eaten mixed into another grain. Use 1 cup grain to 2 cups water and cook for 1 to 2 hours. Cracked wheat has a nutty flavor and cooks in 30 minutes with about 2 cups water to 1 cup wheat. Rolled wheat takes only 20 minutes to cook (2 cups water to 1 cup grain), and is similar to rolled oats. Use rolled and cracked wheat for cookies, breads, or breakfast food. Farina is pieces of endosperm (inner starchy part of the kernel) and usually cooked using 2 to 3 cups water to 1 cup farina for 3 minutes. Pastry wheat is softer and less glutinous and can be used as would other wheat. **NUTRITION:** Whole wheat contains 13 B-vitamins, plus vitamin E, protein, essential fatty acids, trace minerals, iron, and fiber. **STORAGE:** Keep in an airtight container, away from bugs, and in a cool place.

## WILD RICE

Wild rice is actually a grass, not a rice. It has a rounded, hollow stem and flat pointed leaves and grows from 4 to 10 feet high in very wet areas. Tiny flowers with yellow-green blossoms form during July, and the seeds appear 2 to 3 weeks later. The harvesting of wild rice is a tradition among certain Native American tribes in Minnesota. The harvesting is done in late summer. **PREPARATION:** Prepare wild rice as you would other rice. It must be rinsed carefully to remove dust and foreign particles. It triples in volume when cooked. Use 2 1/2 to 3 cups water per cup rice. Try cooking or combining it with brown rice, and use as stuffing, for casseroles, or by itself. It can also be popped like popcorn, doubling in size. Grind it into flour and use in baked goods. **NUTRITION:** Wild rice contains twice as much protein as white rice; it is low in fat and high in the B-complex vitamins. There are more minerals and amino acids in wild rice also.

# SPROUTING MADE EASY

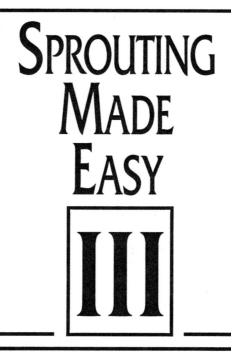

The best way to get fresh, organically grown greens is by growing your own sprouts. Sprouts are low in calories, rich in essential nutrients and chlorophyll, and easy to grow at home.

1. Buy organically grown sprouting material (beans, whole grains or seeds) at a health food store. Place 2 tablespoons of sprouting berries in a wide-mouthed quart container. Fill it with warm distilled water and cover the container with cheesecloth held by a rubber band. Soak overnight.

2. Every morning and evening for the next 3 to 5 days, drain the water from the jar using the cheesecloth as a strainer. Rinse with fresh distilled water, swirling sprouting material around. Drain again, and place the jar in a warm place. Keep the sprouting material moist but not wet or it may rot. If your sprouts dry out between rinsings, top them with a moist white cotton towel or cheesecloth.

3. Harvest sprouts after 3 to 5 days or when they taste best to you.

NOTE: *Mung beans, alfalfa and wheat berries are the easiest to grow but many types of beans and seeds can be sprouted including rye, soy, sunflower seeds and lentils. Each kind has its own unique taste and texture, ranging from sweet to spicy to lettuce like.*

## *The Magic of Fresh Sprouting*

| Type of Sprout | Days Needed to Sprout | Description, Use |
|---|---|---|
| Jumbo sunflower | 10 | Large hardy green leaf. Rich flavor. |
| Black skin sunflower | 10 | Like jumbo sunflower but shells fall off easily. |
| French onion | 14 | Baby onion; absolutely delicious. |
| Garlic chive | 14 | The best way to eat garlic. Chlorophyll reduces odor. |
| Fennel | 14 | Delicious, aromatic, like licorice. For salads and breads. |
| Dill | 14 | Delicious. Great addition to salads and sprout breads. |
| Golden alfalfa | 7 | Hearty mild leafy green for salads or juice. |
| Icicle radish | 6 | Hot, spicy, and colorful. Delicious in salads. |
| Chinese cabbage | 5 | Rich cabbage flavor, small green-leaf salad. |
| Purple turnip | 6 | Sister to cabbage with a great taste. |

| | | |
|---|---|---|
| *Garden kale* | 6 | Another cabbage cousin. Nice, mild flavor. |
| *Brown mustard* | 5 | Very hot! Add to salads. Dry as condiment. |
| *Fenugreek* | 9 | Healthful bitter salad herb. Long stalk and big leaf. |
| *Buckwheat lettuce* | 12 | Long stalk, big leaf, succulent salad green. |
| *Mexican chia* | 14 | Small gelatinous greens. Salad or snack. |
| *Brown flaxseed* | 2 | Two-day sprout makes blended digestive-aid drink. |
| *Shelled sunflower* | 2 | Nutty, healthy, delicious. Great for snacks or salad. |
| *Alaskan green pea* | 5 | Like fresh garden peas. Cooked vegetable or soups. |
| *Mung bean* | 5 | Chinese saute dishes or add to salads. |
| *Adzuki red bean* | 5 | Cousin of mung with flavor. Salad, cook or saute. |
| *Green buffalo lentil* | 5 | Popular addition to salads, soups, sautes. |
| *Red lentil* | 5 | Bright orange cousin of the popular green lentil |
| *Yellow soybean* | 3 | Famous protein-rich super bean. Meaty. Cook, saute. |
| *Garbanzo chickpea* | 4 | Make delicious hummus, soups or side dish. |
| *Red sprout peanut* | 10 | Superb dry roasted snack. Easier to digest. |

| | | |
|---|---|---|
| *Hard red wheat* | *2* | *Sprout breads, crackers, grows wheatgrass.* |
| *Kamut Egyptian wheat* | *2* | *The best sprout bread. Highest protein. Wheatgrass.* |
| *Soft white wheat* | *2* | *Sprout cookies, crackers, cereals, snacks.* |
| *Baker's rye* | *2* | *Delicious sprout breads. Less sweet.* |
| *Sprouting barley* | *2* | *Great sprout breads or high protein wheatgrass.* |
| *Sproutable quinoa* | *3* | *Makes a pretty red grass. High protein.* |
| *Sprouting millet* | *2* | *Snack or grass juice. Light husk, not for cooking.* |
| *Sprouting whole oats* | *2* | *Makes grass juice. Tough husk, not for cooking.* |

# Herbs and Spices: The Source of a Thousand Tastes

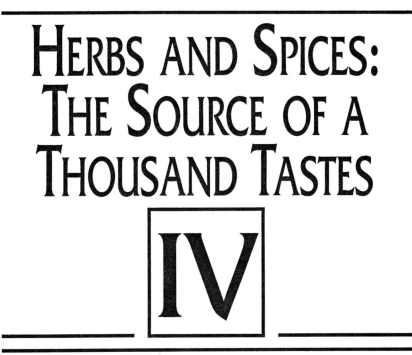

Cooking with spices is an adventure! Just think of ancient times. Explorers would go on long journeys in quest of rare herbs and spices. They would travel over treacherous mountains, high seas, and rugged terrains, battling pirates and thieves. In competition between countries and kings, some nutmeg, cloves or peppers were the motivating force in many of the great exploratory missions to the new world.

Spices are such an important chapter in the history of civilization that today it's possible to distinguish cultures just by the food they eat and the spices they use. Exotic and beautiful places like Goa, Bermuda, and Madagascar are but a few sources of these fascinating flavors. The words "spice" and "spicy" tend to imply an assertive flavor, but skilled seasoning with spices should not be overpowering. We Americans often see spices as little more than salt, pepper, and garlic. However the right blend of spices can be a catalyst for the transformation of simple, plain food into exhilarating cuisine. Your graceful hand, a dash of intuition, and my recipes are just enough spice to enrich the food and captivate your taste buds while your body goes through 30 days of purification and rejuvenation.

*Agar-Agar:* Derived from seaweed, this vegetable substance

often replaces animal gelatin in jams and jellies. When cooking with agar-agar, use 1 tablespoon for very cup of boiling water.

*Allspice:* These dried whole berries may be used in cooking, pickling liquids, and spiced drinks. Ground allspice is a convenient form to use in cooking cakes, pies, and other sweet deserts.

*Anise Seed:* Because it tastes like licorice, anise seed is used in all types of cooking as well as flavoring in beverages. Many people have been known to drink a cup of this soothing tea before going to bed.

*Arrowroot:* An excellent thickening agent, this powered substance makes a good replacement for cornstarch and flour. It is good for thickening gravy, is easy to digest, and has a pleasant taste.

*Basil:* Commonly referred to as sweet basil or garden basil, this classic kitchen spice adds a refreshing warm flavor to foods.

*Bay Leaves:* Also known as sweet bay or noble laurel. Add the tangy taste of these leaves to your soups, stews, and sauces.

*Bee Pollen:* Currently used by athletes as a concentrated source of vitamins, proteins, and enzymes. It makes a great snack or additive to fruit salads or cereals and milk.

*Caraway Seed:* A popular culinary spice used in baking, cooking and salad making. This fragrant seed is also known for the wonderful flavor it adds to tea blends.

*Cardamom:* These delicate seeds are known for the many captivating tastes found in Middle Eastern and Indian sweets and beverages. They are also a tantalizing addition to all types of coffees and cooked dishes, including pies, curries, and vegetable dishes.

*Cassia Buds:* Native to China, this spice is also called Chinese cinnamon. Its luscious taste is reminiscent of both cloves and cinnamon and is a tantalizing addition to deserts.

*Cayenne Pepper:* The name comes from the Greek word *Kapto* "I bite," for it is a biting herb with "fire in the pods." Often called African pepper, this penetrating spice adds a zesty accent to culinary masterpieces.

*Celery Seeds:* A subtle seasoning for soups, salads, and fish dishes.

**Chamomile:** This favorite herb tea is a wonderful after-meal beverage. It is calming when you are tense and soothing to the digestion.

**Chervil:** The name chervil comes from the Greek, meaning "to rejoice" apparently alluding to the fragrance of the plant. Also known as the gourmet's parsley, this aromatic herb of the parsley family is used by chefs throughout Western Europe.

**Chia Seeds:** From the Mexican sage plant, these seeds are used in making teas and in baking bread and muffins.

**Chicory:** This herb is a close cousin of the dandelion plant and is often brewed with dandelion root to make a refreshing beverage.

**Chili Peppers:** These extremely hot peppers add a zesty flavor to soups and sauces. They are an essential seasoning in many Indian, Mexican, and Middle Eastern recipes.

**Chili Powder:** This tangy spice is a pleasing blend of ground chili peppers and other fine herbs and spices. Chili powder is an important ingredient in numerous Mexican-American dishes.

**Chives:** A delicate tasting member of the onion family, dehydrated chives can be used liberally in cooking.

**Cinnamon:** Native to Ceylon, this ancient spice is still one of the most common seasonings used today. Ground cinnamon is used as a spicy sweetener in baking and cooking as well as sprinkled into beverages. Cinnamon sticks are frequently used as swizzle sticks in punches, teas, coffee, wines, and milk, served hot or cold.

**Cloves:** Traditionally used in Chinese courts as a breath freshener, cloves were introduced in Europe by the Arabians and distributed by the Venetians. Today they are utilized in cooking many dishes and spicing numerous drinks.

**Cream of Tartar:** Many recipes suggest using this tart natural fruit derivative in making such things as candies and cake icings.

**Cubeb Berries:** In the ninth century many Arabian physicians used this ingredient to make love potions. Today cubeb berries are predominantly used as a culinary spice; they especially make a good soup seasoner.

*Cumin Seed:* This potent seeds are an essential ingredient in curry powders as well as basic seasoner in numerous Mexican, Indian, and Middle Eastern recipes.

*Curry Powder:* A warm spicy blend of herbs for your favorite East Indian dishes, curry is a must for every serious cook. Medium curry yields a delicious flavor without too much spiciness; hot curry is for those who like to sweat a little while they eat.

*Dandelion Leaves:* This delightful tea also adds a refreshingly tangy taste to snacks and salads.

*Dandelion Root:* The ground roots are frequently roasted and used as a substitute for coffee.

*Dill Seed:* Dill is derived from the old Norse dilla, meaning "to lull." The French use dill seeds for flavoring sauces, cakes, and pastries. Dill is popular in many Middle Eastern dishes and dill seed tea make a restful bedtime tea.

*Dill Weed:* A smoother less pungent tasting version of dill seed, this culinary spice is used in various vegetable, dairy, tofu, and tempeh dishes.

*Fennel Seeds:* These aromatic tasty seeds add a refreshing flavor to herbal and spice blends. In cookery, they can be substituted for dill and anise.

*Fenugreek Seeds:* Whole fenugreek seeds are used in curries in India and as condiment in Egypt. They also make a pleasing and tangy tea.

*Garlic:* Garlic has been praised by many throughout the ages, including the Phoenicians and Vikings who carried large amounts on their sea voyages for added strength and protection. Traditionally known for its zestful flavor in Mediterranean cookery, this favorite culinary spice is now available granulated and minced.

*Ginger:* This popular culinary spice is frequently imported from China and West Africa. It adds a wonderfully robust flavor to all dishes.

*Guaram Masala:* This special blend of aromatic spices is similar to the original Indian blend. Compared to curry powder, it is slightly sweeter and contains no turmeric.

*Kelp:* A sea vegetable that is a high source of such minerals as iodine, iron, and copper. This seaweed accents soups, salads, and breads. In small quantities it may also be used as a salt substitute.

***Leeks:*** Often called spring onions, leeks add an enticing subtlety to sauces, soups, stews, and salads. These leeks are available freeze dried.

***Lemongrass:*** This tasty herb is a frequent ingredient in Thai food and in Indonesian curries. Lemongrass also makes a relaxing tea.

***Lemon Peel:*** This peel is wonderful for cooking and baking and is a good tangy ingredient for potpourris. Use only the peels from organically grown lemons.

***Licorice:*** This ancient Egyptian cure-all is also called liquorice or the sweet root. It is employed by numerous people to relieve their thirst as well as to satisfy their desire for candy, sweets, and cigarettes. Many parents give their children licorice sticks to chew on. Among its various uses, licorice sticks make fantastic swizzle sticks in many drinks.

***Linseed:*** See Flax seed.

***Mace:*** Derived from the outside covering of nutmeg. Mace is a favorite flavoring agent in baking and cooking.

***Marigold Flower:*** Also known as calendula, Marigold flowers can also be brewed into a mild tea as a blood purifier.

***Marjoram:*** The fragrance of this plant gives it its name, which means "joy of the mountain." Sweet marjoram, as it is also called, is an excellent seasoning to keep in stock for cooking a variety of dishes.

***Mustard Seeds:*** This old medicine is often used in poultices. As a cooking spice black mustard seeds are known as an essential ingredient in Indian dishes. The more common variety, yellow mustard seeds, are used in pickling vegetables and making such things as relishes, curries and salads.

***Nutmeg:*** This widely used spice is a wonderful addition to your favorite hot or cold beverage.

***Onion:*** This popular culinary spice is offered in two of the finest forms: ground onion and minced onion.

***Orange Peel:*** A wonderful addition to baked goods as well as in sachets. Orange peel makes a delightful tea. Only use the peel from organically grown oranges.

*Oregano:* An invaluable culinary spice that is an integral addition to most Italian and Mexican dishes. Oregano also makes a stimulating tea.

*Parsley Leaves:* The Greek held parsley in high esteem by crowning their athletic victors with caplets of parsley. Today, parsley leaves are used to garnish and flavor a wide variety of favorite foods, including soups, salads, and meat dishes.

*Pepper:* One of the most popular and important spices used in international cookery.

- *Black Lampong Peppercorns:* These peppercorn from Lampong, India, are available whole or ground.

- *Black Tellicherry Peppercorns:* Reputed to be the finest quality peppercorn available.

- *White Peppercorns:* From Montok, India, these milder peppercorns are available whole or ground.

- *Green Jalapeno Pepper:* A very hot peppercorns used widely in Mexican cookery.

- *Red Crushed Peppercorn:* These spicy peppercorns are commonly used on pizza.

*Poppy Seed, Blue:* A common cooking ingredient. These delicate blue black seeds accent cakes, pastries, breads, and salads.

*Psyllium Seed:* These mucilaginous seeds are used to add bulk to the diet and as stool softeners for those who suffer from constipation.

*Rose Hips:* A good source of vitamin C, many people make a cup of rose hip and hibiscus tea (with a bit of honey) during winter months. Rose hips also add a tangy taste to jams, preserves, soups, and salads.

*Rosemary:* The Latin name Rosmarinus means "dew of the sea." This herb adds a light, pungent flavor for many cooked dishes.

*Saffron:* Considered the gourmet's cooking delight, it has a delicate flavor and adds a golden yellow color to many dishes. It is commonly used in Indian cooking. This delicate spice is hand picked from the stigma of a unique crocus. Approximately forty-three hundred flowers are necessary for each ounce of saffron.

*Sage:* The name comes from the Latin "to be well." A member of the mint family sage is also called red or garden sage. It has been used for centuries both in folk medicine and cosmetically. Today it is a familiar culinary addition to stews, stuffings, sauces, and soups.

*Salt Substitute:* An herbal blend of natural sesame seeds, black sesame seeds, kelp, coriander, thyme, savory, rosemary, basil, caraway, and cayenne.

*Coarse (Kosher) Salt:* A necessity on every spice rack, preferably used in salt mills.

*Savory:* The warm peppery flavor of this well-known kitchen garden plant makes a wonderful seasoning for tofu, tempeh, and vegetable dishes. It is especially flavorful when combined with marjoram and thyme.

*Sesame Seeds:* Popular in Middle Eastern cooking, these tiny seeds are a pleasant addition to any dish. They are available hulled or natural.

*Shallots:* A mandatory ingredient in numerous French recipes, shallots are one of the milder members of the onion family. Shallots add a subtle flavor to soups, sauces, salads, the like. Freeze-dried shallots will last indefinitely (approximately 2 oz. of freeze dried shallots is equal to 1 pound of fresh shallots).

*Spearmint:* A highly stimulating drink, alone or blended with other herds, spearmint adds a delectable freshness to vegetable dishes.

*Tamarind:* This sour fruit is commonly used instead of lemon juice in Middle Eastern, Indian, and Spanish cooking. Soak tamarind fruit before using and make into a refreshing summer or winter beverage.

*Tarragon:* "Little dragon" as it is also named is a delicious culinary herb and an essential ingredient in preparing tarragon vinegar.

*Thyme:* An essential for poultry dishes as well as soups, stuffings, and salad dressings.

*Turmeric:* This spice— an essential ingredient in curry powers and mustards—gives food dishes a golden yellow color. Because saffron is so costly, turmeric is often used as an inexpensive replacement as a coloring agent.

*Vanilla Bean:* This fragrant bean is a popular addition to foods, desserts, and drinks. Brew a pot of coffee with a small bit of a vanilla bean and relax with a delightful tasting drink or try adding broken bits of a vanilla bean to your sugar canister.

# FIVE BENEFITS OF USING HERBS AND SPICES

1. They help to reduce the salt and sugar content of your food.
2. They contain magical purifying properties.
3. They offer high flavor with little or no fat.
4. They're are virtually noncaloric.
5. They create greater variety in your purifying program.

# HEALTHY RECIPES WITH HERBS AND SPICES

## SOUPS

### Vegetable Broth

Vegetable broth can be made by gathering various vegetables (potatoes, carrots, broccoli, string beans, cauliflower, celery, turnips, cabbage, onions, sea vegetables, etc.), cooking them in distilled water in a large pot for about 30 minutes (low flame), and straining the broth. This broth is cleansing and building at the same time.

### Miso Soup

Miso is fermented soybean paste. It has been prized for centuries throughout Asia for its cleansing and healing qualities. Instant miso soup mix can be purchased in most health food stores or you can use miso paste. The paste is mixed into boiling water until it forms a dark broth. Miso is very salty and should be avoided by those who must maintain a low-sodium diet. Miso soup is often served with chopped scallions and small tofu cubes.

### Spicy Garden Vegetable Soup

3/4 cup whole natural sunflower seeds
1 onion, cut into narrow wedges
1/2 cup chopped celery
1 green pepper, cut into slivers
2 tablespoons almond or olive oil
12 oz. Vegebase or vegetable powder mixed in distilled water
1 medium clove garlic, minced
1 teaspoon basil, crumbled
1/2 teaspoon oregano, crumbled
1/8 teaspoon cayenne pepper
1 medium tomato, cut into small chunks

Place sunflower seeds in food processor and process stop-and-go fashion, using steel blade , until coarsely chopped. Bake the onion till soft, place the celery and green pepper in the vegetable broth, with garlic, basil, oregano, and cayenne pepper. Heat through. Add tomato and heat through. After the fire is turned off mix in oil. Ladle into soup bowls. Spoon sunflower seeds into centers of bowls. Makes 4 servings, about 1 1/4 cups each.

## E-Z ABC Soup

1 cup whole wheat alphabets
3 cups water
Small piece bay leaf
1/2 teaspoon onion powder
1/4 teaspoon garlic powder
1 teaspoon olive oil
2 tablespoons soy sauce
1 teaspoon dried parsley or soup herbs

Bring water to a boil with bay leaf, onion and garlic powders, and oil. Add alphabets and simmer for 8-10 minutes until done, adding soy sauce and herbs during last few minutes. For extra body and protein, reheat some cooked beans in this soup while it's simmering, or boil chunks of tofu along with the alphabets. Sprinkle with a little Parmesan cheese or nutritional yeast, if desired. Makes 2 to 4 servings.

# YOUR HOME GUIDE TO JUICING

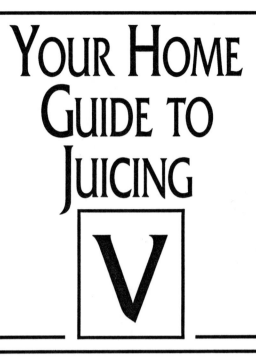

## PREPARING FRUITS AND VEGETABLES FOR THE BLENDER

Fruits and vegetables need only washing and cutting up. If organically grown, no peeling is necessary, if bought in a regular market, then washing and peeling are recommended. Celery will blend smoothly, including strings. If using hot broth, any vegetable or cooked beans or grains can be added.

1. Start the blender about 1/4 or 1/3 full of liquid.
2. Cut the vegetables and fruits into chunks and add them slowly while the blender is on. (This might save you getting a chunk of something hard, like a carrot, stuck in the blades.)
3. Keep the mixture thick, adding more liquid as it thickens.
4. For a smoother consistency, add a banana or ice cubes or both. Ice also cools the drink and makes it more appetizing.
5. Pour into serving pitcher and thin with juice to taste.

**GETTING THE MOST OUT OF YOUR BLENDER DRINKS**

Add any of the following for a refreshing, nutrition rich, body purifying beverage.

Fresh vegetables of any kind, (carrots, celery, beets, cabbage,
asparagus, etc.)

Fresh fruits of any kind (bananas, apples, oranges, peaches,
grapes, etc.)

Raw and unsalted nuts and seeds (walnuts, pecans, sunflower,
pumpkin, etc.)

Unsulfured, unsweetened dried fruits (dates, raisins, apricot,
etc.)

# NUTRITION-RICH BREAKFAST ELIXIRS

1. Start with the liquid you want to use. Some of the most popular are

   Unsweetened frozen pineapple juice concentrate

   Tomato juice

   V-8 bottled juice (only if you cannot make fresh juice)

   Papaya

   Unsweetened grated coconut

   Nut and seed milks made by blending nuts and seeds with
   distilled water

   Apple cider
2. Fill the blender about 1/4 full of juice or liquid.
3. Place a layer of something soft like cabbage pieces.
4. Add pieces of carrot, beet and apple and blend. To get it as
   smooth as possible, keep it thick.
5. When everything you want to add seems to be as smooth as
   possible, add a banana and some ice cubes; add more
   pineapple juice if mixture is getting too thick.

**MY FAVORITE BLENDED RECIPES**

16 oz. pineapple juice

1 large beet or 2 or 3 smaller ones, cut up

1 large carrot or more smaller ones, cut up

1 or 2 Jerusalem artichokes (sun chokes), pieces of celery, parsley, etc.

1 banana and ice cubes.

Start with 1/4 blenderful and keep adding ingredients till thick. This recipe should be sweet enough with the pineapple juice and banana, but add a few teaspoons of honey, maple syrup, or barley malt syrup if you want.

## APPLE CRANBERRY PUNCH

1/2 cup either fresh or frozen raw cranberries

1/2 cup honey

1 cup water

1 apple, unpeeled and quartered

Blend the mixture until it is thick and smooth. Strain through a wire strainer, shaking and stirring the mixture to keep it straining. Don't rub it through the strainer too hard in order to keep the punch clearer.

Add enough water to make about a quart of punch. This will still be strong enough so you can add ice to the punch bowl. Repeat and make as many batches as you need for your punch bowl.

You can serve the cranberries left in the strainer as a relish either alone or mixed with nuts, grapes, pineapple, and so on.

## HOMEMADE V-8

2 cups canned tomatoes

1/2 to 3/4 cup celery pieces or tops

1 piece of cabbage

1 wedge of romaine or Boston lettuce

1 piece of onion or onion top

1/2 cup carrot pieces

1 teaspoon vegetable seasoning (such as Vegebase; available in your health food store)

1 large size sprig of parsley

1 piece of sweet red or green pepper.

Blend the mixture until it is thick and smooth. Add ice cubes at the
end to cool it and make it smoother. Sprinkle in some lemon juice or
spices to add zest. Generally, the taste will be similar to the canned
V-8 juice you buy.

## ALTERNATE INGREDIENTS FOR THE HIGH-PROTEIN FRUIT SMOOTHIE

*Fresh peach:* Use 1/4 cup honey, 1/2 teaspoon almond flavoring and 4 medium peaches.

*Fresh apricot:* Same as peach using 7 unpeeled, halved apricots.

*Red fruits (cranberry, strawberry, raspberry):* Use 1 cup
unsweetened fruit plus 5 tablespoons honey.

*Dark fruits (blueberries, etc.):* Use 1 1/2 cups of fresh fruit
and vanilla flavoring, and 5 tablespoons honey.

*Yellow- or orange-colored fruits:* Use 1 cup fresh fruit and
almond flavoring, alone or with vanilla, plus 5 tablespoons
honey.

*Papaya juice:* Use 1 cupful in place of fruit plus 5 tablespoons honey.

You can adjust the amount of honey you add to suit your taste.

## CITRUS SPLASH

3 tablespoons sunflower seeds
1/4 cup orange juice
1 cup-lowfat milk
6 ice cubes

Mix all the ingredients in a blender for 1 minute or until smooth.
Makes 1 serving.

## TROPICAL QUENCHER

1/2 cup pineapple chunks
1/2 banana (sliced)

1 cup low-fat milk

6 ice cubes

Mix all the above in a blender for 1 minute or until frothy. Makes 1 serving.

## SUNSPICE SMOOTHIE

1/4 teaspoon cinnamon powder

1 cup plain yogurt

1/4 cup apple chunks (diced)

Mix yogurt and apple pieces well; add cinnamon, place in a freezable dish and allow to become firm. Mix well and enjoy. Makes 1 serving.

## BERRY HEAVEN

3 tablespoons blueberries (fresh or unsweetened frozen)

2 tablespoons strawberries (fresh or unsweetened frozen)

4-5 tablespoons raspberries (fresh or unsweetened frozen)

1 cup low-fat milk

6 ice cubes

Mix all the ingredients in a blender for 1 minute or until smooth. Makes 1 serving.

## HIGH-PROTEIN FRUIT SMOOTHIE

2 cups of unsweetened frozen fruit (see suggestions)

1 cake of soft tofu

1 teaspoon vanilla

Blend well and add 1 cup ice cubes or until thick. Blend the mixture until thick.

# CLEANSING TONICS, ELIXERS, AND POTIONS

1. Start with the liquid you want to use. Some of the most popular are

Unsweetened frozen pineapple juice concentrate
Tomato juice
V-8 bottled juice
Papaya
Unsweetened grated coconut
Nut and seed milks made by blending nuts and seeds with
distilled water
Apple cider

2. Fill the blender about 1/4 full of juice or liquid.
3. Place a layer of something soft like cabbage pieces
4. Add pieces of carrot, beet, and apple and blend. To get it as
   smooth as possible, keep it thick.
5. When everything you want to add seems to be as smooth as
   possible, add a banana and some ice cubes; add more
   pineapple juice if it is getting too thick.

## FLUSHING TOXINS OUT OF YOUR LIVER

As your body is purifying the liver plays an important role in the
process. It is for this reason that the liver must be specifically
cleansed as well. One of the most effective ways for doing this is the
Liver Flush.

### THE LIVER FLUSH

Every morning prepare a liver cleansing tea consisting of:

l teaspoon of olive oil
1/2 teaspoon of fresh chopped or grated ginger
l teaspoon fenugreek (a seed found in health food stores)
Juice of one whole lemon
1 pinch of capsicum (cayenne pepper).

Take 1 cup of boiled distilled water, letting it cool for 1 or 2 minutes.
Add these ingredients (add the olive oil when you are ready to drink
it). Strain the mixture and drink the remaining liquid. If you wish,
you can put the entire mixture in a blender and drink the liquefied
ingredients. Although some people may find the taste unusual, it is a

powerful cleanser for the liver, the digestive tract, and the intestines.

This is a modified version of a "liver flush" developed by Doctor Randolph Stone, a well-known physician and authority on natural medicine.

# LEWIS HARRISON'S 25 FAVORITE JUICE FORMULAS

## THE HEALING POWER OF ENZYMES

One of the most important aspects of fresh juice therapy is the amount of enzymes that they make available to the system. Plant food enzymes are extremely valuable on all levels of the healing and rehabilitation process. According to N. Walker, a pioneer in the use of juice therapy in the United States, "The juices extracted from fresh raw vegetables and fruits furnish all the cells and tissues of body with the elements and the nutritional enzymes that they need, in the manner to which they can be most readily digested and assimilated" (*Raw Vegetable Juices*, p. 13, by N. Walker, Pyramid Books). These are my favorite enzyme-rich formulas.

| #1 | apple | 8 oz. |
|----|-------|-------|
|    | beet | 5 oz. |
|    | carrot | 8 oz. |
|    | cucumber | 5 oz. |
|    |       |       |
| #2 | carrot | 8 oz.. |
|    | celery | 8 oz. |
|    | parsley | 8 oz. |
|    |       |       |
| #3 | carrot | 10 oz. |
|    | cabbage | 3 oz. |
|    | celery | 3 oz. |
|    |       |       |
| #4 | cabbage | 6 oz. |
|    | cucumber | 6 oz. |
|    | grapefruit | 4 oz. |

(not recommended in colitis)

| #5 | carrot | 14 oz. |
|----|--------|--------|
|    | horseradish root | grate 1/2 teaspoon of this root into the carrot juice |
|    | lemon juice | 1/2 lemon squeezed |

| #6 | apple | 8 oz. |
|----|-------|-------|
|    | beet | 5 oz. |
|    | carrot | 8 oz. |
|    | cucumber | 5 oz. |

| #7 | apple | 4 oz. |
|----|-------|-------|
|    | beet | 2 oz. |
|    | carrot | 4 oz. |
|    | celery | 4 oz. |
|    | spinach | 2 oz. |

NOTE: *Those who suffer from kidney stones should remove spinach from this juice combination.*

| #8 | alfalfa sprouts | 2 oz. |
|----|-----------------|-------|
|    | beet and beet tops | 2 oz. |
|    | carrot | 6 oz. |
|    | celery | 6 oz. |

| #9 | asparagus | 5 oz. |
|----|-----------|-------|
|    | carrot | 2 oz. |
|    | cucumber | 5 oz. |
|    | kale | 2 oz. |
|    | pear | 2 oz. |

| #10 | carrot | 4 oz. |
|-----|--------|-------|
|     | cucumber | 10 oz. |
|     | raw potato | 2 oz. |

| #11 | carrot | 7 oz. |
|-----|--------|-------|
|     | green pepper | 5 oz. |

| #12 | carrot | 7 oz. |
| | cucumber | 6 oz. |
| | parsley | 2 oz |

| #13 | brussels sprouts | 5 oz. |
| | carrot | 2 oz. |
| | escarole | 7 oz. |
| | string beans | 5 oz. |

| #14 | carrot | 6 oz. |
| | celery | 3 oz. |
| | escarole | 7 oz.. |

| #15 | beet | 2 oz. |
| | carrot | 4 oz. |
| | cucumber | 6 oz. |
| | parsley | 3 oz. |

| #16 | carrot | 10 oz. |
| | dandelion | 3 oz. |
| | turnip leaves | 3 oz. |

| #17 | carrot | 6 oz. |
| | spinach | 3 oz. |
| | turnip leaves | 3 oz. |
| | watercress | 4 oz. |

| #18 | grapefruit | 4 large or medium size |
| | lemon | 3 medium size |
| | distilled water | 3 quarts |

This formula, which is a modification of a formula used by N. Walker, is used to realkanilize the body and cleanse the lymphatic system. It is best used over a two- to three-day period as part of a fast. Approximately 6 oz. is taken every 30 minutes until the entire mixture has been taken. At the end of the day, take a glass of celery/carrot combination. At the end of the three days begin the raw food program described in Chapter 5.

| #19 | carrot | 7 oz. |
| | celery | 4 oz. |
| | parsley | 2 oz. |
| | spinach | 3 oz. |
| | | |
| #20 | carrot | 10 oz. |
| | spinach | 6 oz. |
| | | |
| #21 | beets | 4 oz. |
| | carrot | 6 oz. |
| | celery | 4 oz. |
| | cucumbers | 6 oz. |
| | | |
| #22 | carrot | 6 oz. |
| | celery | 6 oz. |
| | spinach | 6 oz. |
| | | |
| #23 | carrot | 8 oz. |
| | celery | 6 oz. |
| | cucumbers | 2 oz. |
| | | |
| #24 | carrot | 16 oz. |
| | celery | 16 oz. |
| | | |
| #25 | beet juice | 8 oz. |
| | green leafy | |
| | vegetable Juice | 8 oz. |
| | dandelion juice | 1 oz. |

In addition to juice formula recommendations, Purification Tea can be taken throughout the day.

## COFFEE, TEA, COCOA, AND ALCOHOL

Avoid coffee! There are many reasons for this recommendation but the main one is the caffeine and other naturally occurring chemicals in this beverage. These chemicals include theophyline, theobromine, and methylxanthine. Don't become disheartened. There are a number of safe and healthy alternatives to high caffeine beverages. Here are a few alternatives.

## Coffee Substitutes

There are many pleasant-tasting coffee substitutes in supermarkets and health food stores. If you have been a long-time coffee drinker, you will find that these may take some getting used to, but there is a solution to this dilemma. Rather than eliminating coffee altogether, you can start out with 50 percent of each and slowly decrease the coffee. In a few weeks time you should be 100 percent coffee free.

## Tea

In recent years the choices of caffeine-free teas has expanded to a point where you could probably drink a different flavor every day for a month. There are also some caffeine-free pekoe teas, and these are acceptable though herbal tea such as chamomile, peppermint, or other choices are superior.

## Cocoa

It is unfortunate that cocoa contains caffeine and theobromine because chocolate treats like chocolate milk and hot chocolate are very popular with small children. Chocolate is also very high in fat, which is one of the reasons that it has such a smooth, rich texture. In recent years many people have begun to replace cocoa and chocolate with a wholesome and tasty powder made from the carob fruit. Carob has much less fat and sugar than cocoa derived products and is higher in fiber as well. Here is a recipe for a carob beverage that can be taken hot as a replacement for cocoa or cold as a shake:

## Hot or Cold Carob

> 2 tablespoons carob
> 1/4 cup sunflower oil (olive oil would have too strong a taste for this recipe)
> 6 cups of nonfat dry milk or goat's milk*
> 4 teaspoons of honey (or barley malt syrup)*
> 4 teaspoons vanilla

Both goat's milk and barley malt syrup are available in health food

Dissolve the carob powder in oil, add a little milk, and heat the mixture for a few minutes to cook the carob. Place the mixture in a blender with the rest of the ingredients until it is smooth. Serve hot or refrigerate. This yields 4 to 6 servings.

## Alcohol

Alcoholic beverages tend to be high in calories and low in other nutrients. Even moderate drinkers may need to drink less if they wish to achieve ideal health.

On the other hand, heavy drinkers may lose their appetites for foods containing essential nutrients. Vitamins and mineral deficiencies occur commonly in heavy drinkers — in part, because of poor intake, but also because alcohol alters the absorption and use of some essential nutrients.

Sustained or excessive alcohol consumption by pregnant women has caused birth defects. Pregnant women should limit alcohol intake to 2 oz. or less on any single day.

Heavy drinking may also cause a variety of serious conditions, such as cirrhosis of the liver and some neurological disorders. Cancer of the throat and neck is much more common in people who drink and smoke than in those people who don't.

# HOME DOCTORING WITH JUICES, HERBS AND SUPPLEMENTATION

# VI

Many people who use the 30-Day Body Purification Program have specific health problems that require special supplements, homeopathic remedies, juice formulas and herbs. The baffling array of treatments for the relief of various health problems can result in frustration and expense in a search for a medical "cure" that may not yet exist. In addition, there is often no one treatment that works for everyone. For these reasons, therapies focusing on diet, stress-reduction, vitamins, amino acids and exercise are gaining popularity.

While dietary management is often the only treatment some people need for their health problems, others may require intensive medical intervention. *The following suggestions are not designed to replace competent medical care where necessary.* Some of the remedies listed here are folk remedies that have been used successfully for many years. Many are well-known through published scientific research. All of them are included here to help you heal your body both during and beyond the 30-Day Body Purification Program.

# HOW TO USE THIS SECTION

**It is best to use the suggestions offered in this section under the guidance of a a skilled consultant or a wholistic or nutritionally trained physician.** Some of the information provided is derived from scientific research while much of it is based on folk remedies or the authors own experience. The best thing to do is to experiment with different approaches within the general structure of the *30-Day Body Purification Program.*

# HOME DOCTORING TOOLS

- Supplementation - This may include vitamins, minerals, amino acids, or other nutritional products available in a capsule, pill, powder or liquid form.
- Herbs - This may include the leaves, roots, oils, alkaloids, seeds, barks, flowers or fruits of various trees or plants. These are usually available a capsule, pill, powder or liquid form. The liquids usually consist of an extract based on alcohol, water, glycerine or apple cider vinegar or a combination of these extracting agents.
- Tissue Salts - These are homeopathically prepared ( a unique process where remedies are administered in extremely dilute dosages) remedies. They were developed by Wilhelm Heinrich Schuessler, a German Physician in the 19th century. According to Schuessler these remedies (there are twelve different ones) eliminate deficiencies of the vital inorganic elements that are essential to life.
- Aromatherapy - Aromatherapy uses the oil based essences of plants. These oils evaporate at room temperature and have a distinctive aroma. They generally work in through one of five ways; as a

  1. Stimulant
  2. Sedative
  3. Antiseptic
  4. Anti-spasmodic
  5. Anti-inflammatory

- Juice Therapy - A juice extractor is required for the preparation of these formulas and combinations. If not directed otherwise each formula you use should be taken twice daily (morning, and evening.) If possible use organically grown fruits and vegetables. If this is not possible remember to peel off the skin. All Formulas are listed in the Appendix by #.
- Hydrotherapy - This includes full body baths, foot and hand baths showers and compresses (herbal teas, or mashed herbs wrapped in a cloth and placed on an area of the body.)

# REMEDIES FOR 180 COMMON HEALTH PROBLEMS

## ABSCESS

- Supplementation - Supplements that you can use to help reduce the effects of this condition include vitamin A, B complex, C, and E. It is important to increase your water intake to at least 8 glasses a day.
- Herbs- Try red clover tea or golden seal extract. A warm baked onion compress will help open a hot swollen abscess
- Tissue Salts - A combination of the following may be of help:

  1. Early stage -Ferr. Phos
  2. Swelling but no pus -Kali Mur.
  3. To open abscess - Silicea
  4. Final stages - Calc. Sulph.

- Aromatherapy - Place the aromatic oil of Garlic on a new or not highly inflamed abscess.

## ADENOIDS

- Juice Therapy - Try a combination of carrot/spinach juice.

## ADDISON'S DISEASE

- Juice Therapy - Try a combination of romaine lettuce juice with a small amount of powdered sea kelp added. Beet/celery/lettuce is also a popular combination.

**NURIA**

- Aromatherapy - Inhale the aromatic oil of Juniper.

## ALCOHOL USE AND ABUSE

Alcoholic beverages are high in calories, low in nutrients and contain many undesirable additives. Also, alcohol use is directly responsible for a loss of vitamin C in the body, and this loss of vitamin C may contribute, in turn, to other nutritional deficiencies.

Not surprisingly, alcoholics are commonly lacking in vitamin C, zinc, and magnesium. Further, alcoholics may have difficulty absorbing thiamine, folic acid, and vitamin $B_{12}$. As a result they may be predisposed to hypoglycemia, chronic fatigue, adrenal insufficiency, headaches, ulcers, cirrhosis of the liver and other health problems.

The first step on the road to recovery from the effects of alcohol is to cleanse the system of toxins. The 30-Day Purification Program will rid the body of metabolic wastes, toxins, and other poisonous substances accumulated through the use of alcohol. A week of juice fasting will also provide enzymes which are valuable to the healing and rehabilitation process. Be aware that all fasts beyond 2 to 3 days should be conducted under the supervision of a health professional familiar with the benefits and limitations of fasting programs.

- Juice Therapy - Under supervision fast on juices for 10 to 14 days. Try formula #18. It can can be included among the juice mixtures that are especially healthy. Or you can squeeze ten lemons in two quarts of water; drink a glass every two hours. Another helpful drink is a mixture of seven ounces of green leafy vegetable juice and seven ounces of beet juice combined with two ounces of dandelion juice. Take this combination twice daily.

## ALLERGIES

In addition to simplifying your diet and eliminating allergenic factors; begin a juice therapy program. Twice a day, drink this 18-ounce mixture -12 ounces of carrot juice, 3 ounces of beet juice, and 3 ounces of cucumber juice.

What are allergies? According to *Taber's Encyclopedic Medical Dictionary* an allergy is "An altered reaction of body tissues to a specific substance (allergen) which in nonsensitive persons, will, in similar amounts, produce no effect."

An allergic reaction results because the body identifies this food or substance as an intruder, as a potentially dangerous attacker, and then reacts to the intrusion. Though allergies are antibody-antigen reactions, there are cases where the body reacts much as it would in a typical allergic reaction although no antibody can be isolated. These are often called sensitivities by those who suffer from them. Researchers believe that in these cases, the reaction may be due to the release, from injured cells, of a body chemical called histamine.

For example many people react to meat, eggs, and milk products. As soon as the protein combines with a certain antibody in their blood, the body mounts a counterattack by producing the chemical histamine. It is this chemical histamine, that causes the typical symptoms of allergic reactions, such as swollen blood vessels, inflamed skin, tightened air passages, and itching of the eyes. All this discomfort for what is essentially a "false alarm"! For many people the symptoms of allergy and sensitivity are quite similar.

Recent studies show that allergy-like reactions and problems are not limited to foreign substances—known as allergens—combining with antibodies alone. Allergens may also react with other blood elements. Add to this the fact that there are many more conditions caused by allergies and food sensitivity that are not recognized as such, and you begin to see the scope of the problem. In fact, allergic reactions may be the most frequently unrecognized cause of illness in the United States!

## Disorders Associated with Allergies

Many disorders are actually symptoms resulting from allergies or certain sensitivities. It is for this reason that the elimination of certain foods from the diet or the addition of certain spices may be so useful in helping many seemingly unrelated disorders.

*Among the disorders whose symptoms can be tied to allergic or sensitivity responses are:*

- anemia
- arthritis
- bloating
- bursitis
- canker sores
- chills

- circulatory problems
- coughing
- cramps
- dandruff
- depression
- EKG changes
- headaches
- heart pain and palpitations
- hearing and ear problems
- hoarseness
- hyperactivity
- inflammation
- joint pain and swelling
- fatigue
- menstrual difficulties
- nosebleeds
- rectal pain and itching
- urinary problems
- vaginal itching and burning
- vision and eye problems

- vomiting
- wheezing
- gastrointestinal disorders
- flatulence
- colitis
- colic
- nausea
- diarrhea
- ulcers
- respiratory disorders
- asthma
- respiratory disorders like bronchitis, pneumonia
- skin disorders like contact dermatitis, itching, eczema, rashes, hives & welts.
- Weak adrenal gland function.
- Low digestive enzymes and poor nutrient absorption.
- Photosensitivity to drugs and chemicals.

## Diagnosing Your Allergies

There are several methods for diagnosing your allergies. The most common and most effective are described here.

THE FOUR-DAY FOOD-ROTATION PLAN. Following this plan, as the name broadly hints, you eat a particular food in modest amounts every four days. As you do so, keep a detailed diary of (1) which foods you eat; (2) when you eat each food item; (3) how much you eat of each item; and (4) your reactions, if any, to each food, even seemingly insignificant reactions.

In this way, you can better isolate specific symptoms, associate the reactions with certain foods, and then avoid those foods. Although this method for identifying food sensitivity is obviously inexpensive, it is not as accurate as other procedures. To improve its accuracy, this plan is often used together with Dr. Coca's Pulse Test. [Arthur F. Coca, The Pulse Test, New York: Lyle Stuart, 1967.]

RAST. The radioallergosorbent test, simply known as RAST, is an inhalant test that determines antibody levels for specific allergens that might be present in your bloodstream. RAST not only identifies which inhalants cause allergic responses but also shows the degree of severity of each response. Therefore, it is especially helpful in identifying the appropriate treatment. RAST results are more specific than results from cytotoxic testing.

CYTOTOXIC FOOD TESTING. In this lab test, a doctor or technician uses a blood sample to test the reaction of your blood cells to 150 (or more) different foods. Using a microscope, the doctor or technician determines your allergy to foods by observing how severely each food destroys white blood cells.

### The First Two Weeks:

Many foods, including many common foods, can cause allergic reactions. Thus when you begin the first two weeks of the 30-Day Body Purification program you should eliminate those foods which are the top ten offenders including:

| | | |
|---|---|---|
| Wheat | Corn | Most Dairy products* |
| Eggs | Nuts | Seafood |
| Chocolate | Alcohol | Citrus fruits |

* Unflavored yogurt, Kefir and buttermilk as well as goat's milk are acceptable.

### KEEP THIS IN MIND

Care during infancy. Breast-fed children have fewer allergies than bottle-fed children. Also, if infants are fed highly antigenic foods (such as cow's milk and eggs) during the first few months after birth, then food sensitivity is likely to develop, especially if the infants have a hereditary disposition toward allergies.

Acidophilus (lactobacillus acidophilus) is a bacterial strain that has numerous healing properties, especially concerning the immune system. High-potency strains of acidophilus (1) build strong immunities, (2) maintain intestinal acid balance, and (3) inhibit the growth of unfriendly bacteria in the urinary tract, as well as in the respiratory and reproductive systems. In addition to its specific usefulness in fighting allergic reactions, acidophilus is a very useful, general healing tool. Acidophilus is especially recommended when you are taking antibiotics.

*NOTE: If you have a milk allergy, begin taking acidophilus in very small doses and monitor any reactions you may have. Better yet, use an acidophilus product cultured from a non-milk source.*

## A Four Week Supplementation Program

To reduce the effect of food sensitivity, you may find the following program useful. Though it may seem like a large amount of pills and powders it will be worth it:

• Supplementation:

**One hour before mealtime take:**
1 level teaspoon of sodium ascorbate powder (vitamin C)
3 to 5 100-milligram bromelain tablets (A digestive enzyme product)
Approximately 15 milligrams of free form amino acids

**With your meals:**
100 to 250 milligrams of vitamin $B_6$ (pyridoxine)
Five 100-milligram tablets of $B_2$ (riboflavin) throughout the day
500 milligrams of pantothenic acid

## Additives in Supplements & Drugs:

Many drugs as well as nutritional supplements that are designed to treat allergy symptoms contain certain ingredients either in the tablet coating or the tablet itself which may actually aggravate the condition. Among these ingredients are:

Dyes, coloring agents and artificial flavors
Preservatives (in tablets, usually benzoates)
Sulfates (for example, ferrous sulfate)
Binders, fillers, lubricants, coatings and inert substances
Coal tars

Sugar, starch, salt
Animal-derived stearates and pesticide residues

When buying supplements, focus on those that contain no yeast, wheat, soy, corn, or dairy.

When buying bread crumbs chose a wheat free variety.

## ALZHEIMERS

A Harvard University researcher has found that cigarette smokers are up to 4 times as likely to get Alzheimers disease as people who don't smoke. This is one more reason to quite smoking

## AMBLYOPIA

Supplementation - Vitamin $B_1$ is the primary nutrient used to correct this condition. In addition to $B_1$, vitamin B complex, and vitamins A, C and E can be used as supportive nutrients.

## ANEMIA (iron deficiency)

Nutrition - Eat foods rich in iron. Iron rich foods are especially effective in combating anemia. The following foods are all good sources of iron. Fruits: apples, apricots, bananas, dark grapes, strawberries. Vegetables: alfalfa, beets, broccoli, carrots, kale, onions, okra, potatos, radishes, spinach, squash swiss chard, tomatoes, watercress, yams.

Other Iron-rich foods include sunflower seeds, black beans, peas, and crude unsulfured blackstrap molasses.

At the same time avoid caffeinated beverages. Caffeine interferes with the body's ability to absorb iron. Increases in your intake of protein will also help Anemia.

- Juice Therapy - Enjoy any of the following freshly pressed vegetable and fruit juices:

| | | |
|---|---|---|
| Alfalfa sprouts | Carrots | Swiss chard |
| Beets | Kale | Tomatoes |
| Broccoli | Spinach | Watercress |
| Fruits | Plums | Dark grapes |
| Apricots | Strawberries | |

For juice recipes that are especially helpful in fighting anemia, see Juice Therapy Formulas #8, 17, and 19.

## APHONIA

- Juice Therapy - Try juice formula #20

## APOPLEXY

- Juice Therapy - Try formula #8, #19

## ARTHRITIS

- Nutrition - Many foods are perfectly acceptable for arthritic patients, but certain foods have demonstrated special healing powers and therefore deserve close attention. While on the Purification Program use plenty of potassium broth and add sea vegetables such as dulse, hiziki, wakamae, and kelp. Seaweed also provides an abundance of vitamins and minerals.

Other key foods and juices are:

Cherries and cherry juice.

Fresh fruit and vegetables

Raw potato juice (do not use if you have rheumatoid arthritis)

Parsley, alfalfa, watercress, string beans, wheat grass and garlic

Wheatgerm oil (one tablespoon per day)

Blackstrap molasses -unsulfured (one tablespoon per day)

People who suffer from arthritis should pay special attention to the value of nutritional therapy.

### *Avoid the following foods:*

Refined breakfast cereals

Canned foods

Roasted nuts and seeds

Anything with hydrogenated fats or oils (read package labels carefully!)

Alcohol

Coffee and tea

White rice, white flour and white sugar

Jams and jellies

Soft drinks

Meats

# FOLLOW THESE DO'S AND DON'TS FOR RELIEF FROM SPECIFIC TYPES OF ARTHRITIS PAIN:

## GOUT

Avoid foods high in purines, including organ meats, bouillon, gravy, yeast, and certain fish (particularly anchovies, herring and sardines).

Eat cherries (either fresh or frozen) or drink cherry juice. Cherries are especially valuable in fighting the symptoms of gout.

Lose weight, but do not begin your diet while you are suffering from an acute gout attack. Dieting can increase the uric acid in your blood.

## RHEUMATOID ARTHRITIS

Avoid chicken, fish, grains, liver, and potatoes. Removing fats and oils from your diet and cutting sodium intake to a minimum is essential.

For pain relief, try these three simple steps; (1) follow a vegetarian diet( no meats, Poultry, fish, and eggs); (2) avoid coffee, tea, alcohol, and strong spices; and (3) supplement your vegan diet with vitamin $B_{12}$.

Raw food diets can be very effective for arthritis. Avoid most dairy products but be sure to add fermented dairy products such as yogurt, buttermilk etc. Fruits which are helpful are lemons, grapes, plums, black currants, grapefruit, apricots, cherries and blackberries. Also add to your diet these important greens: parsley, alfalfa, watercress, string beans and mung bean sprouts.

Beware of dietary programs that promise an "arthritis cure". Many of these programs tell you to avoid certain foods—for example, citrus fruits- that supposedly cause acid intoxification, which in turn, further aggravates arthritis symptoms. Certain arthritis sufferers may indeed have sensitivity to citrus fruits. However, oranges and other citrus fruits are know to have an alkaline effect on the system and in certain situations may actually assist the healing process.

- Juice Therapy - This approach is especially effective in treating the symptoms of arthritis. Always use freshly pressed juice, not canned or bottled juice.

See Juice Therapy Formula #8, 21, 22, 23 and 24.
If you suffer from gout, here is an especially helpful formula.

- Add four ounces of distilled water to twelve ounces of cherry juice.
- Drink this mixture for relief from gout pains.

Many nutritional consultants believe that the enzyme bromelain, which is found in pineapples, reduces swelling and inflammation in different kinds of arthritis.

## ASTIGMATISM
- Juice Therapy - Try Juice therapy formula #6, 14, 17.

## ATOPIA
- Supplementation - Take Evening Primrose Oil, an excellent source of EFA's (Essential Fatty Acids).

## ATHLETES FOOT
Honey spread on area and then covered with gauze will bring relief. One can also rub the itchy area with ice cubes for relief. Tea Tree oil has also been found to be affective for relief from this condition.

- Supplementation - Some vitamins which are useful for athletes foot are A, C, and E. Make sure to change your socks every day. Dust feet with garlic powder to ease rashes.

## AUTISM
- Supplementation -There have been some reports that amino acid and megavitamin supplementation can support improvements in those autistic children whose condition is not resultant from disease of the brain. Among the nutrients that may be beneficial are the following: glutamine, vitamin B complex, vitamin $B^6$ (450 mg daily), vitamin C (1 - 3 gm daily), Niacin (1 - 3 gm daily), and Pantothenic acid (200 mg daily). This program should be introduced under the guidance of a competent health professional. Nutrients given in therapeutic amounts should always be administered by a professional trained in nutrition.

## BAD BREATH
Colonization of putrefying bacteria in large numbers in the throat,

tongue and mouth causes halitosis (bad breath). When these putrefying bacteria are dominant in the intestine, they produce objectionable gases. Acidophilus helps keep the bacteria in check, thus helping prevent bad breath.

You can purchase the lactose digesting enzyme in the form of a product called Lact-Aid. Lact-Aid can be purchased in some health food stores or by writing to Sugerlo Company, 600 Fire Road, P.O. Box 111, Pleasantville, NJ 08232. Make sure you brush your teeth after every meal and floss daily.

## BALDNESS

This is generally not a health problem as much as it is an image problem. Causes may include genetic factors, aging, hormonal changes, nutritional deficiencies and emotional stress. Stress-induced and deficiency-induced baldness may be eased with supplementation. Special attention should be given to the following:

- Supplementation - Increase intake of vitamin B complex, B2, B6, C, E Biotin, choline, folic acid, inositol, niacin, PABA, pantothenic acid, Bioflavonoids, and the mineral copper.

Some additional corrective methods for baldness are:

- Juice Therapy - Try a combination of carrot/beet/spinach.
- Herbs - Use horsetail, fenugreek, chamomile, rosemary.

## BED WETTING

There does not seem to be a consensus on the specific cause. Hidden food allergies are often considered the culprit. RAST allergy testing is recommended. The most common food allergens in bed wetters are milk, wheat, eggs, corn, citrus, and tomatoes. Any food, however, may prove to be the culprit. Musculoskeletal problems, especially abnormal curvature of the spine, might also cause or aggravate the problem. Spinal adjustments as well as general massage and bodywork have been found to be helpful in many cases. Infants and children under 2 should not be given any herbs or nutrients by mouth, unless under professional supervision.

For problems with bedwetting, try the following;

- Supplementation - Vitamins A, C, B complex, calcium, magnesium.

- Herbs - Use extract or tea of oat straw, juniper berries or plantain. Hypnosis has been successful in treating this condition.
- Juice Therapy - Try Juice Therapy Formula #6.
- Tissue salt - Take Kali. Phos., especially for nervous high strung children.
- Hydrotherapy - Try walking in cold water and/or upper body sponging.
- Emotions - According to the many healers, there are many misconceptions among parents and health professionals concerning bed wetting, which, if not addressed will only add to the child's confusion and lower self esteem. Wet pajamas and sheets pose no threat of disease since urine is bacteria free. It may not even be necessary to change the child's pajamas or bed cloths when he/she wets. Many children do not experience any physical discomfort after bed wetting. It may in fact be a warm and pleasant sensation, even reviving unconscious memories of earlier life. It is important for parents not to over react to bed-wetting while addressing the situation appropriately.

## BELL'S PALSY

Chiropractic or osteopathic manipulation is very effective here. As for supplements try Vitamin B complex, vitamin C, vitamin $B^1$ and $B^{12}$ injections.

- Supplementation - Increase your intake of Vitamin A.

## BITES (ANIMAL)

See a physician immediately if you are bitten by a wild animal or if your own pet has been allowed to run free and might have been bitten by a rabid animal.

- Aromatherapy -Use oils of lavender and sage applied topically.

## BLADDER DISORDERS

It is valuable to use foods high in lactobacillus acidophilus such as homemade yogurt and buttermilk. Many bladder disorders manifest as a burning sensation while urinating. Take one tablespoon of apple cider vinegar in eight ounces of distilled water each morning until the burning subsists. Continue using this combination for five more days. To reduce pain of a bladder infection, add catalyst altered water to regular drinking water.

- Juice Therapy - Add a small amount of onion or garlic to Juice Therapy Formula #6. Drink 8 ounces of cranberry juice three times per day. This will acidify the urine and reduce bacterial activity that may be causing the bladder infections. Watermelon juice by itself is also very helpful.

## BLOOD BUILDING

Increasing intake of the following nutrients will help to build up the blood:

- Supplementation - Increase your intake of vitamin B12, folic acid, C, and the mineral iron.
- Herbs - Use rhubarb root.
- Juice Therapy - Drink beet juice to help to build new red corpuscles.

## BODY ODOR

After proper tests to eliminate physical causes try the following:

- Supplementation - Increase your intake of calcium and magnesium, PABA (para-amino-benzoic acid), zinc, liquid chlorophyll, and acidophilus.
- Herbs - Spread lemon juice under the arm pits and other odorous areas. Apply baking soda or corn starch to underarms to absorb and neutralize strong odors. Some individuals have a fishy smelling body odor because of a possible defect in their ability to metabolize trimethylamine, a substance produced by certain foods that are high in choline. Among these foods are eggs, fish, liver, and beans (especially soybeans). When eating of these foods is avoided the situation usually clears up (Journal of Pediatrics, June 1979). Witch hazel, Arnica lotion, calendula and coriander extract are all natural astringents which have a tendency to close the pores of the skin. These herbs also have antibacterial properties which may be helpful.

## BRAIN FUNCTIONING

- Supplementation - Increase your intake of Niacin, L-Glutamine, Niacin, vitamin $B_1$, choline, inositol, pantothenate, cysteine, RNA, and the mineral phosphorus. All of these nutrients have all been shown to improve brain function.

## BROKEN BONES

Get plenty of sunlight, calcium, vit. D, and Homeopathic Arnica.

## BRUISING WITHOUT APPARENT CAUSE

This involves the rupture of tiny blood vessels. The condition may be associated with obesity, anemia and the menstrual period.

- Supplementation - Increase intake of vitamin B complex, folic acid, vitamin D, iron, bioflavonoids, rutin, bromelain, hesperidin, calcium, silica, vitamin C, and vitamin K.
- Hydrotherapy - Use ice packs and cold water soaks to treat bruises resulting from a contusion.

## BURSITIS

Try these treatments:

- Supplementation - Increase intake of vitamin A, B complex, and vitamin E. Vitamin $B_{12}$ injections can be administered by a physician or taken orally by placing 1,000 mcg under the tongue each day. Make sure to take extra Vitamin C as an anti-inflammatory agent.
- Herbs - Apply a hot comfrey or flax seed poultice after the initial stages.

Ask your physician about trying TENS Therapy(a type of electrical, muscular stimulation) and ultrasound therapy. Both of these have been shown to reduce pain and inflammation.

## BUERGER'S DISEASE

- Supplementation - Some useful supplements are vitamin E (up to 2,400 iu), lecithin, AND vitamin C.

## CALLUSES

- Supplementation - When not formed as a natural protection for the skin, vitamin A deficiency may be indicated. Along with vitamin A, other helpful supplements include vitamin D, vitamin E, chlorophyll and safflower oil.

## CANCER

*The 30-Day Purification Program* can eliminate many carcinogenic factors from your body. You already know the general value of fresh vegetable and fruit juices. For a patient who is not too weak, a fast of raw fruits and vegetables may be helpful, but the fast should be short, only two or three days at the most.

In Europe and Canada, many naturopathic physicians recommend Biota Brand beet juice as well as an herbal formula known as Essiac. Both are available in many American health food stores.

In addition, try these juices:

- Mix the juice from carrots, spinach, and beets.
- Drink the juice of beet crystals.
- Mix carrot juice with black cherry juice.

Remember to use only fresh products for your juices.

Increase your intake of cruciferous vegetables (cabbage and cauliflower, for example), whole grains, beans and high carotene foods such as carrots, collard greens, spinach, cantaloupe, beet greens, broccoli, apricots, papaya, prunes, peaches, watermelon, and squash (yellow, zucchini, butternut, acorn and hubbard). Also include strawberries and tomatoes. These seem to have cancer preventing properties as well.

Take four tablespoons of pureed asparagus daily. Beans are another food which should be eaten regularly. They contain a protease inhibitor which may block cancer.

Reduce the amount of fat in your diet to no more than 20 percent of your total caloric intake. To do so, avoid or drastically cut your intake of vegetable oil, margarine, meat, and poultry. If you do eat poultry, remove the skin. Also, cut your intake of high-fat dairy products which include whole milk, sour cream, butter, cream cheese and other cheeses.

Do not eat foods that have been smoked, pickled or barbecued. They contain carcinogens.

Avoid foods which contain nitrates and nitrates, additives commonly found in deli meats, bacon, and smoked fish. These additives react with the body's amines to form nitrosamines compounds, which may cause cancer. If you do eat these foods occasionally, increase your intake of vitamin C. Vitamin C interferes with the formation of nitrosamines.

Avoid frying or broiling meats. The process of frying or broiling produces at least eight chemical mutagents that may contribute to certain types of cancer! Instead, learn to steam, boil, bake, pressure-cook, stew and poach your foods.

## CANDIDIA ALBICANS

- Nutrition- Increase your intake of The most effective nutritional program to combat Candida albicans is a yeast-free, low carbohydrate diet. Avoid baker's yeast and any baked goods that might contain it (for example, alcoholic beverages.)

Also, be sure to avoid refined sugars, vinegar, relishes, mushrooms, aged cheeses, dried fruits, and fruit juices. Eat plenty of fresh vegetables, sea vegetables, grains, beans, and a small amount of fresh fruit.

High-potency supplements of Lactobaccilus acidophilus have been confirmed in clinical studies to be effective in treating Candidiasis, and have been shown to restore the beneficial intestinal environment. Vaginal or rectal application of acidophilus in a yogurt base has also been effective. Lactobacillus organisms are normal constituents of vaginal flora. They contribute to the maintenance of the acid PH by fermenting glycogen in the mucous to lactic acid. It should be noted that yogurt has long been used as a folk remedy for vaginitis. An anthroposophical doctor I know recommends reducing the intake of beans and increasing the intake of foods high in lactic acid such as buttermilk and sauerkraut. She says that the lactic acid creates an body environment hostile to Candida.

## CANKER SORES

These sores usually appear in the lining of the mouth or on the tongue. Sometimes they are a form of Herpes Simplex. At other times, they can be an indication of digestive problems.

- Supplementation - Medical studies indicate than many people who suffer from recurrent, canker sores also have deficiencies of iron, folate and/or vitamin $B_{12}$. Supplementation with these nutrients resulted in a remission from the sore (Journal of the American Medical association February 12, 1982). Other useful nutrients include vitamin A, B complex, $B_1$ niacin, C and D formula, 300 - 1,500 mg. of lysine daily until they disappear, acidophilus and high acidophilus yogurt. Apply vitamin E oil directly to the sore. Take folic acid.
- Edgar Cayce recommended Ipsab. Place an ice cube directly on the sore in the early stages for the best relief.
- Herbs - Apply witch hazel, camphor spirits or myrhh extract directly on the sore with cotton rinsing your mouth with diluted hydrogen peroxide may reduce or eliminate the symptoms. Burdock root is another effective herb.

## CARBUNCLE

- Supplementation - Increase your intake of vitamins A, C, D, and E.

## CARDIOVASCULAR DISEASE

- Nutrition - Increase your intake of add plenty of soy products to your diet, such as, soy grits, tofu, tempeh, and soy beans. Soy protein is effective in lowering blood cholesterol. Also eat walnuts and seaweed. Like soy, walnuts and seaweed contain omega -3 fatty acids, which may be responsible for lowering blood cholesterol.

Eat plenty of legumes, including these dried beans: black beans, kidney beans, lentils, chick peas, lima beans, and split peas.

Add black tree fungus to your diet. This edible fungus (known as "mo-er"), which commonly is used in Chinese cooking, has anti-clotting properties that may account for the low rate of heart attacks in China. Specifically, this fungus contains adenosine, an anti-clotting agent also present in garlic and onions.

- Juice Therapy -

  For angina, try Formulas #8 and #19.

  For arteriosclerosis, try Juice Therapy Formula #20. Red grape juice may be a helpful addition to your diet.

Acidophilus possesses anti-cholesteremic and anti- lipidemic factors for reducing cholesterol. Several studies show significant reduction of serum cholesterol levels after supplementation with Acidophilus.

- Supplementation - Increase intake of vitamin E, co-enzyme Q10, and carnitine.

## CATARACTS (A CLOUDING OF THE LENS OF EYE)

A reduction of riboflavin and vitamin C in the lens of the eye has been found to be a possible contributing factor to the development of cataracts. Studies have indicated that many individuals who have cataracts and are under the age of 50 have levels of certain chemicals in their blood indicating that they are carriers of a genetic disease called Galactosemia. Galactosemia is generally treated by eliminating all dairy products from the diet. A few researchers believe that this dietary approach seems to retard the progress of cataracts in carriers and possibly even cause them to shrink. According to the same researcher, foods rich in riboflavin have a protective effect against cataracts (A report in the *New York Daily News*, Monday, June 21, 1982 on the work of Dr. Harold Skalka, Chairman of Ophthalmology at the University of Alabama). Some preliminary studies indicate that there may be some connection between cataract formation and selenium deficiency. Eyes with cataracts usually have much less selenium than is found in normal eyes. Increase intake of Vitamin $B_2$.

## CERVICAL DYSPLASIA

- Supplementation - Supplementation with folate may reverse mild varieties of this condition in women who take birth control pills. Vitamin A & C may help build resistance.

## CHICKEN POX

Increase caloric intake and vitamin A and C if there is fever. Use

- Tissue Salts - A combination of the following may be of help:

1. Take Ferr. Phos. hourly at onset of fever.
2. During eruptive period Ferr. Phos. should be alternated with Kali. Mur. hourly.
3. Take Kali. Sulph. to reduce scaling of the skin.
4. Take Calc. Phos. during convalescence. Trim fingernails to reduce scratching.

## CHOLERA

- Aromatherapy - Inhale the aromatic oils of cinnamon, eucalyptus, peppermint, or sage.

## CIRCULATORY PROBLEMS

- Tissue Salts - A combination of the following may be of help:

1. Take Calc Sulph 6X (tissue salt) to cleanse the blood.
2. For poor circulation use a tissue salt combination of Calc. Flour., Calc Phos., Kali Phos., and Mag Phos..

- Juice Therapy - Drink parsley juice for maintaining the integrity of the capillaries and arterioles.
- Aromatherapy - Inhale the aromatic oils of cypress, lavender, sage, and thyme orally in combination (see directions for use under aromatherapy).

## COLIC (ABDOMINAL GAS IN CHILDREN)

Give infants sips of warm peppermint or fennel tea and apply heat to abdomen. If you are feeding the child cow's milk, switch to goat's milk. Doctors have also found a connection between drugs given to the mother during labor and colic in their babies. The indiscriminate use of drugs can cause colic in babies (*Journal of the American Academy of Pediatric* 62.402, 1978)

## COLLAGEN DISEASE

- Herbs - Take green barley juice powder and slippery elm bark tea or extract.

## CONJUNCTIVITIS

- Supplementation - Special attention should be given to vitamins A and $B_6$. Also take extra vitamin B complex, niacin, and vitamins $B_2$, C, and D.
- Aromatherapy - Inhale the aromatic oils of chamomile and lemon dispersed through the room. Place a cold compress on eyes (see hydrotherapy).
- Tissue Salt - Take Ferr. Phos.

## CONVALESCENCE

- Tissue Salt -After an illness, Calc. Phos. (tissue salt) will aid assimilation and tonify the entire system.
- Aromatherapy - Inhale the aromatic oils of lemon, sage and thyme.

## CROUP

See the program described in the entry on Respiratory Disorders.

## CUSHING'S DISEASE

- Supplementation - Supplementation with potassium may help to this problem.

## CYSTIC BREAST DISEASE

- Supplementation - Vitamin E can reduce the effects of this condition,
- Nutrition - It is important to avoid coffee, tea, cocoa or chocolate and all other products and beverages containing caffeine.

## CYSTIC FIBROSIS

• Nutrition - Try switching to a high protein, low fat diet. The recommended diet is 25% higher in calories than a normal diet. These extra calories are taken in the form of protein rather than fats since those afflicted with this condition have poor digestion and absorption of nutrients. Malnutrition even on a normally healthy diet is always a potential problem. Some studies have indicated symptomatic benefits to afflicted children when their diets were supplemented with corn oil, vitamin E and pancreatic enzymes. Increase also the intake of vitamin A, B complex, sodium, and vitamins C, D, E, and K. Increase vitamin K for some afflicted infants. Massage, swimming and other aerobic exercise will help keep lungs clear of mucus. Some experimental studies have indicated that periodic infusions (oral supplementation did not seem to make a difference) of soy oil resulted in the improvement in one of the biochemical abnormalities of the disease in children. It is theorized that the high linoleic acid content of soy oil makes the difference. It has been shown that Cystic Fibrosis patients have abnormally low blood levels of this Essential Fatty Acid. All therapies should be applied under a physician's guidance.

## DENTAL AND ORAL PROBLEMS

• Juice Therapy

For healthy teeth try Juice Formula #16 (see Appendix V) or a combination carrot and other vegetable juices.

For pyorrhea, drink one pint of spinach juice daily. Limit your use of fruit juices.

Remember to brush and floss regularly.

## DERMATITIS HERPETIFORMIS (CLUSTERS OF ITCHING OR BURNING SKIN LESIONS)

Eliminate gluten from the diet. For further information see entry on skin disorders.

## DIABETES MELLITUS

If you have diabetes, you will find the following combinations health building.

- Juice Therapy
- Drink one pint of string bean juice each day.
- Try Formula #13 (see Appendix).
- Mix and drink the juice of carrots and Jerusalem artichokes (which actually belong to the sunflower family, not the artichoke family). According to N.W. Walker, considered by many to be the pioneer of juice therapy, Jerusalem artichokes contain a starch-like substance that does not require insulin to be digested by the body.
- Drink cucumber juice. It may contain a plant hormone that helps the pancreas produce insulin.

## DIGESTIVE DISORDERS

- Juice Therapy - For all gastrointestinal disorders, you may take Formulas #1 and #4 . In addition, you may drink fresh papaya, wheatgrass, pineapple, or lemon juice. If you wish, you can mix whey with your juices, or you can buy Biota brand juices, which already contain whey.

Here are some juice remedies for specific conditions:

- For Amoebic Dysentery: Drink garlic juice.
- For Colitis: Drink papaya juice and raw cabbage juice. Also, follow the juice program for ulcers, listed next. Avoid citrus juices.
- For Ulcers: Combine 12 ounces of carrot juice with 4 ounces of cabbage juice and drink the mixture once a day for one week. After one week, slowly increase the amount of cabbage juice in the mixture from 4 to 12 ounces.

Also mix raw potato and cabbage juice and drink the combination immediately after extraction otherwise the mixture loses the healing value of vitamin U.

- For Constipation and Ulcers: Five times a day, drink 3 ounces of celery juice mixed with 3 ounces of cabbage juice. Also, each day drink 1 pint of spinach juice, the most powerful juice for relieving constipation.

- For Sluggish and Prolapsed Colon: Drink sorrel juice, which is available at Jamaican food stores.
- Acidophilus produces enzymes which help digest food and decrease bloating.
- For Dizziness and vertigo: Take the tissue salt Kali Phos 6x. Have your physician check for any infections or injuries of the inner ear. Other possible causes include anemia, brain tumors, irregularities of blood pressure, emotional stress, nutritional deficiencies (especially vitamin $B_6$ or niacin), lack of oxygen and low blood sugar.

• Supplementation - Supplements to increase are vitamin B complex, choline, niacin, inositol, vitamin C, vitamin E and calcium.

## DIAPER RASH

Try catalyst altered water on the irritated area. The rash should clear up within 24-48 hours. Use disposable diapers instead of cloth or rubber. Avoid the use of excessive soap or alcohol when changing diapers. Spread zinc oxide cream and vitamin E oil on the infected area. Avoid talc. Use cornstarch as powder instead.

## DUPUYTREN'S CONTRACTURE

Take 800 IU-1200 IU vitamin E daily.

## EDEMA (WATER RETENTION)

Try increasing vitamin B6 and taking these herbs in tea or as extracts: corn silk or parsley root.

• Juice Therapy - Drink formula #5,
• Tissue salts - take Nat.Mur (tissue salt) 6x, and try a low sodium diet.
• Aromatherapy - Inhale the aromatic oils of garlic, onion, geranium.

## ENDOMETRIOSIS

- Nutrition - Increase your intake of protein by using more fermented milk products and grain and bean combinations.
- Supplementation - Supplements you can use to help reduce the effects of this condition are B vitamins (especially choline & inositol), selenium, Vitamin C and Vitamin E.

## EPILEPSY

- Nutritional Conditions - A special diet called a ketogenic diet has been found effective in controlling epilepsy in children 2-5 years of age. This diet consists of an unusual ration (4:1) between fats, carbohydrates and proteins. It is believed that this diet which may consist of large amounts of high fat foods such as butter, cream, sour cream, cream cheese etc, somehow control epileptic attacks by increasing the level of ketones (products of fat digestion) in the body. (Pediatric research Vol 14, No 12, 1980). This diet should be supplemented by thiamine and B vitamins as well as other vitamins and minerals to reduce the potential side effects of the diet itself. (British Journal of Opthamology, No. Vol. 63, No. 3,1979.) A ketogenic diet should be administered only under medical supervision.
- Supplementation - GABA (Gama Aminobutyric Acid), vitamins A, B complex, $B_6$, $B_{12}$, C, D, E, folic acid, calcium pangamate, pantothenic acid, calcium, magnesium, manganese. Research conducted by Dr. Yukio Tanaka of St. Mary's Hospital in Montreal, Quebec, Canada "has demonstrated a link between manganese deficiency and convulsions in humans. He also states that pregnant women with a deficiency of magnesium may give birth to epileptic children." (Nutrition Almanac, Nutrition Search Inc. McGraw Hill Pub. p.134) Epileptic convulsions respond in many cases to vitamin $B_6$ supplementation (*Journal of Nutritional Science and Vitaminology*, Vol.25, No 5, 1979), magnesium, manganese, choline, folate, and Vitamin D.

- Aromatherapy - Inhale the aromatic oils of basil, cajuput, rosemary, thyme, chamomile.

- Emotions - In addition to the more common grand mal and petit mal types of epilepsy there is a form of the condition known as temporal lobe epilepsy which seems to respond well to Behavioral Therapy.

## EYE AILMENTS

- Juice Therapy - Drink a combination of carrot/green pepper/parsley juice.
- Herbs - Drink a tea made from eye bright.

## FAINTING

- Aromatherapy - Inhale the aromatic oils of cinnamon and rosemary in a steamer, burnt in a candle, or in a massage oil.

## FLEAS

- Aromatherapy - Inhale the essence (aromatic oil) of turpentine.

## FEVERS

Fevers below 101° F should not be of concern. Aspirin is not recommended by most physicians, especially for children since its use in children with chicken pox or influenza has been identified as a cause of a disease called Reye's Syndrome. (Pediatric News, Vol 16, No.4 1982. For fevers above 102° F use the following remedies:

- Drink plenty of fluids to offset the loss of water.
- Wrap yourself in a wet cotton bed sheet or constantly have yourself sponged with cool water.

- Supplementation - Increase intake of Vitamins A, $B^1$, C, D, & E, calcium, magnesium and phosphorus. Sodium and potassium should be replaced since this is easily lost from the perspiration accompanying the fever.
- Hydrotherapy - take a ginger oil bath while keeping cool packs at the base of the neck.

- Aromatherapy - Inhale the aromatic oils of eucalyptus, hyssop, lavender or sage to steam or massage oil.
- Herbs - White willow bark extract or tea are the best choices. Other herbal remedies include sage, echinacea, garlic, cayenne pepper, yarrow, ginger tea, ginger oil or tea added to the bath, vervain and elm bark (usually in the form of lozenges).
- Tissue Salts - Ferrum Phos. 6X is a quick remedy often used in high fevers. Use Kali sulph 6X to promote perspiration and keep a fever from rising too high.
- Hydrotherapy - Take a basin of water filled with ice water and place your hands in the basin intermittently for 20-30 minutes.

## GALLBLADDER PROBLEMS

- Juice Therapy - Juices is an important approach to keeping your gallbladder functioning properly.
- Drink 3 pints daily of Juice Therapy Formula #6.
- Squeeze one fresh lemon and add the juice of 6 ounces of hot distilled water. Each day, drink 6 to 10 glasses of this mixture.

## GANGLION

- Hydrotherapy - Try a high pressure cold shower directly on the ganglion.

## GANGRENE

Hyperbaric Oxygen Therapy (this must be done under physician's supervision) has been found very helpful in reducing diabetic gangrene. It is helpful if the patient is given vitamin E during this treatment.

## GLAND PROBLEMS OF A GENERAL NATURE

- Juice Therapy - Try carrot and asparagus juice in combination.
- Aromatherapy - Place a few drops of the aromatic oils of cypress, garlic, onion or sage on the skin in the area where

the glands are located. Some acupuncturists may place similar essences on acupuncture points for the glands in question as a part of their treatment. Increase intake of Vitamin A, B complex and C.

## GLAUCOMA

Avoid tobacco, alcohol, coffee and tea.

- Supplementation - Vitamins and supplements that you can use to help reduce the effects of this Increase Vitamin B complex since the accompanying symptoms of stress may be connected to a deficiency of these vitamins. Vitamins for general eye health: 60-250 mg. vitamin C per pound of body weight, Rutin, vitamin A, choline and pantothenic acid.
- Juice Therapy - Drink plenty of lemon, grapefruit, orange, carrot and beet juice each day.
- Herbs : Hemp (marijuana) has been shown to reduce the pressure that glaucoma produces. At this time it can only be obtained under doctors prescription and is the subject of great controversy between the patients who require it and the the United States Governments anti-drug policies.

## GOITER

- Supplementation - Iodine is the key nutrient to help reduce the effects of this condition. This should be done under a physician's guidance. Key support nutrients that you may want to increase your daily intake of include vitamin A, C, and the mineral calcium.

## GROWING PAINS IN CHILDREN

Take 200 I.U. of Vitamin E daily until the pain disappears. Avoid refined foods, and increase your intake of whole grains, and raw and unsalted nuts and seeds. Wheat germ oil will also be helpful in reducing the pain..

- Aromatherapy - Apply the aromatic oils of lemon or onion while massaging the child's aching limbs or have child breathe in the the aromas via a steamer or an aromatherapy diffuser.

## GYNECOLOGICAL DISORDERS

- Juice Therapy - Try the following recommendations:

- For Amenorrhea: Drink Juice Therapy Formula #15.
- For General Menstrual Problems: Try a combination of beet, carrot, and fennel juices. Drink dark fruit juices — grape, prune, cherry, and black currant are enriching for blood circulation.
- For Premenstrual Syndrome (PMS): Drink the juices of watermelon, cucumber, asparagus, and parsley.
- For Vaginal Infections: Add 2 teaspoons of liquid chlorophyll to each serving of carrot juice three times a day.

## HAIR (ALSO SEE BALDNESS)

Most hair loss is due to naturally occurring genetic factors and should not be viewed as a health problem. Other causes of hair loss may include: hormone imbalances, general stress, nutritional deficiencies (especially protein, B vitamins and zinc), allergy triggered by stress (this type of baldness is known as alopecia areata), hair follicle destruction (this can be a result from X-ray overdose, burns, chronic hair pulling, certain types of cancer, certain rare skin diseases such as lupus erythematosis and scleroderma.) Ringworm and viral infections can also cause hair loss.

For these individuals the following suggestions may be of help.

- Juice Therapy - Drink a combination of equal parts of cucumber and green pepper juice.
- Tissue Salts - A combination of the following may be of help: Try a combination of Kali Sulph., Nat. Mur., Silicea and Silicea 6X.
- Herbs - Jojoba is said to help to restore color to gray hair.
- Supplementation - Supplements that you can use to help reduce the effects of this condition include PABA, pantothenic acid, folic acid, brewer's yeast) and blackstrap molasses and L-Cysteine. L-Cysteine is the most plentiful amino acid in human hair and is essential for maintaining and growing healthy hair.

## HALITOSIS (BAD BREATH)

The causes of this condition can include poor diet, gum disease, infections of the nose or throat, gum conditions, tonsillitis, sinusitis, anemia, tooth decay, excessive smoking or a high bacterial count in the mouth. Avoid excessive intake of carbohydrates.

- Supplementation - Supplements that you can use to help reduce the effects of this condition include vitamin C which is essential for healthy gums, and vitamin A, $B_6$, B-complex, C, niacin, and the mineral zinc. other valuable supplements include alfalfa or chlorophyll tablets, betaine HCL and whey powder.
- Edgar Cayce's Formula - Try Ipsab gum treatment formula as a rinse for your mouth after eating.
- Nutrition - Reduce your intake of cooked foods and increase your use of fresh vegetables especially the green leafy ones. Be sure to avoid sugar and refined carbohydrates. They help to feed bacteria in your mouth that can increase unpleasant odors.

### Personal Care:

- Floss your teeth and massage your gums regularly.
- Chew a piece of gum after your meals. recent studies indicate that gun chewing reduces the buildup of plaque in the mouth. (choose a sugar free health food store brand).
- Eat parsley or chew on cloves.
- Make a mouthwash of 1 tsp. powdered myrrh, 1/2 tsp. liquid chlorophyll and two tablespoons. of warm water.

- Aromatherapy - Inhale the aromatic oils of nutmeg, peppermint, rosemary and thyme. eliminate antibiotics. (Holistic Health Digest, Vol. 34, May/June 1985).

NOTE: *Acidophilus capsules can reduce extremely foul breath caused Candida Albacans. See chapter on Candida)*

## HEEL SPURS

Change your diet so that you lose weight. This will reduce the pressure on your heels. It is also helpful to place a foam pad in your shoe to reduce the pressure.

## HEMORRHOIDS

This is a type of varicose vein that may be caused by a diet low in fiber, pregnancy and/or bearing down too hard during a bowel movement (constipation or diarrhea is known to aggravate this condition).

- Supplementation - Supplements that you can use to help reduce the effects of this condition include vitamin E, B-complex, and C. Other value supplements include rutin, the amino acid methionine, bioflavonoids, and the minerals calcium and magnesium.
- Herbs - Use extracts or teas of butcher's broom, bayberry root, witch hazel, shepard's purse or yarrow. Adding raw miller's bran and other high fiber foods to your daily diet was shown to help this condition according to a report in a scientific journal. ("Disease of the Colon and Rectum", Vol. 25, No. 5, 1982)
- Juice Therapy Therapy - A popular juice therapy for eliminating hemorrhoids is a combination of carrot, spinach and turnip juice with a small amount of mustard green and celery juice added. Juice therapy formula #17 also works well.
- Tissue Salts - A combination of the following may be of help: Take a combination of Calc. Flour., Calc. Phos., Kali Phos. and Nat. Mur.
- Hydrotherapy - Take alternating hot and cold sitz baths. Warm chamomile sitz baths may be helpful and soothing.
- Aromatherapy - Inhale the aromatic oils of cypress, garlic and onion. Take classes in postural training and movement reeducation so that you will put less stress on your abdominal and back muscles, as it is this stress that may contribute to hemorrhoidal discomfort. Drink plenty of fluids to keep your stools soft. Avoid refined foods. Insert a suppository from peeled garlic bud or raw potato. Use *The 30-Day Purification Program strictly!*

It is also important to cleanse the liver. For an effective liver cleansing:

1. Use teas or extracts of the following herbs: Oregon grape root, goldenseal and dandelion root.
2. Increase your fiber intake by using more whole foods such as beans and grains. These tend to soften the stools. Psyllium seed husks and flax seeds are also recommended as additions to your diet.
3. Soothe and heal the irritated hemorrhoidal tissue. Collinsonia or stone root is an herb that has been found to have this effect If you cannot obtain Collinsonia root, try the following herbs: plantain, witch hazel, cransebill, comfrey or mullein. Several of these herbs contain tannin which is known to have a powerful astringent effect. This can reduce the hemmorhoidal tissue.

## HEMORRHAGING (ABNORMAL BLEEDING FROM ANY PART OF THE BODY)

- Tissue Salts - A combination of the following may be of help: If there is bleeding from a wound use Ferr. Phos. applied as a powder locally. Increase the use of cayenne pepper in your diet.
- Supplementation - Bioflavanoids are a supplement that you can use to help reduce the effects of this condition.

## HICCUPS

Many home remedies work on the principle of creating a counter-irritant that will force the phrenic nerve into a coordinated rhythm.

- Aromatherapy - Inhale the aromatic oil of Tarragon.
- Supplementation - calcium is a mineral that you can use to help reduce the effects of this condition.

Other popular treatments that have been used to reduce or stop hiccups include taking a deep breath and holding it as long as possible, then blowing out slowly; drinking a glass of water in one gulp; swallowing dry bread or crushed ice; putting pressure on the eyeballs, and placing an ice bag or heat on the diaphragm (just below the rib cage).

## HOOKWORM

- Aromatherapy - Inhale the aromatic oil of thyme or thuja.

## HOSPITAL INDUCED NUTRITIONAL DEFICIENCIES

- Supplementation - Researchers have found that meals served in hospitals may be low in the minerals copper and zinc. It is important to supplement theses minerals if you will be confined to a hospital bed for some time (research reported in *J. Amer. Med. Assoc.*, May 4, 1979).

## HYPERACTIVITY IN CHILDREN

Many nutritionally oriented physicians believe that most hyperactive children are strongly affected by hypoglycemia, allergies, or vitamin, mineral and/or enzyme imbalances. Eliminate all artificial colors and flavors from the diet including those in vitamins and medications (do not eliminate medications without competent supervision). Eliminate tomato products, pickles, and cucumbers as well as any foods that are high in salycilate (aspirin-like) compounds including almonds, apples, apricots, berries, cherries, grapes, raisins, raspberries, oranges, cucumbers, nectarine, peaches, plums and prunes. Eliminate all foods that have been generally shown to aggravate a hyperactive condition including milk, corn, wheat and eggs as well as all refined sugar. (*Journal of Learning Disabilities*, May 1980). Children love ice cream but are usually prohibited from having it on this dietary program. Ice Bean, a non-dairy frozen dessert available in most health food stores, is acceptable according to the Feingold Foundation approval list. Ice Bean is available in many health food stores..

- Supplementation - Supplements that you can use to help reduce the effects of this condition include giving the child large amounts of vitamin C, B complex, $B_6$, Niacin, Pantothenate and essential fatty acids. This was reported to be effective in an article in the magazine *Medical Hypothesis*, May 1981. High dosages of nutrients should be given to children only under the supervision of a nutritionally trained physician.

Recommended Reading - *Why Your Child Is Hyperactive* by Ben F. Feingold, M.D., Published by Random House, 1974.

## HYPERTENSION

Limiting your sodium intake is usually the first step to reducing high blood pressure. Sodium is an essential nutrient, but excessive amounts of sodium may contribute to high blood pressure. Sodium causes fluid retention, and excess fluid adds stress to the heart and the circulatory system.

One teaspoon of table salt contains 2,000 mg. of sodium. According to the National Research Council an adult can safely take about 1,100 to 3, 300 mg. of sodium daily. Some estimates show that the average American adult now consumes from 2,300 to 6,900 mg. of sodium daily! Thus, you must monitor your sodium intake carefully; not an easy chore, because sodium may be scattered throughout your diet.

Do you add salt to your foods at the table? If salt has been added to your foods during the processing or during the cooking, then you are adding additional salt. To eliminate salt as a food additive, avoid these foods:

Baking soda and baking powder, salty fish, sodium nitrate & sodium nitrite, most snack foods, Monosodium glutamate (MSG), desserts, most cheeses (unless labeled salt-free), Tamari, Meat (especially processed meats), Shoyu, Pickles, food containing soy sauce, olives.

How do you start? Read the labels on food packages. Labels that claim "low sodium" will specify the sodium content. Generally, however, unprocessed fresh foods have much less sodium than any processed packaged food. To reduce sodium intake at mealtime, learn to use lemon juice, apple cider vinegar, cayenne pepper, and onion or garlic powder instead of prepared sauces and high salt condiments. When you're in a restaurant look for the low sodium selections on the menu!

- Avoid Caffeinated Beverages - Studies show that even a few cups of coffee ( or its equivalent) can raise your diastolic blood pressure an average of 14 percent-within one hour.

- Juice Therapy - Drink parsley juice for maintaining the integrity of the capillaries and arterioles.

- Many nutritionists consider juicing to be the most efficient method for lowering systolic pressure. For best results, use Juice Therapy Formula #12 for two to four weeks. If this is too concentrated, try several one-week-long Juicing programs over a period of about six months.

In addition to Juice Therapy Formula #12, you can also use all citrus juices as well as watermelon, beet, cranberry (unsweetened), spinach, and grape.

- Try the Watermelon Diet: Try a diet of only watermelon for one week. NOTE: Do not attempt this diet if you have diabetes or hypoglycemia.

Perhaps the high potassium content of the foods in a raw food diet are responsible for the radical lowering of blood pressure in hypertensive people who switched to such a diet?

Foods high in potassium content that are recommended :

| | | |
|---|---|---|
| Orange juice | Apricots | Avocados |
| Potatoes | Lima beans | Tomatoes |
| Squash | Bananas | Peaches |

Eat plenty of onions. Onions contain prostaglandin-Al, a hormone-like chemical that lowers blood pressure.

## HYPERTHYROIDISM

- Supplementation - Supplements that you can use to help reduce the effects of this condition include vitamin A, B complex, C, and E. Other beneficial nutrients include choline inositol, and the minerals calcium and iodine. Thyroid problems require proper diagnosis and medical supervision.

## HYPOTENSION (LOW BLOOD PRESSURE)

Symptoms of this condition can include slow heart rate, dry skin, hair loss, scanty or no menstrual flow, fatigue, excessive sleepiness, abnormal weight gain, poor memory, puffy hands and constipation. This condition may sometimes be the result of allergies (especially eggs, wheat, rice, potatoes, caffeine and yeast).

- Supplementation - Supplements that you can use to help reduce the effects of this condition include iodine, zinc, kelp, vitamin C, and E. It may also be helpful to add a tablespoon of extra- virgin olive oil to your salads daily.
- Herbs - Drink teas made with the following herbs: golden seal, bayberry, myrrh, or black cohosh. If you are unable to do so then buy them in extract from in your local health food store.
- Aromatherapy - Inhale the aromatic oils of camphor, hyssop, rosemary, sage and thyme.
- Juice Therapy - Try Juice formula #17 or Juice formula #6.

## IMMUNE-SYSTEM DISORDERS

The juices listed below are excellent tonics for strengthening the immune system.

| | | |
|---|---|---|
| Carrot | Orange | Green pepper |
| Black currant | Garlic | Watercress |
| Lemon | Beet | Pineapple |

## IMPETIGO

- Supplementation - Supplements that you can use to help reduce the effects of this condition include vitamins A C, D and E. Also use garlic oil, squeezed from capsules onto the affected area.

## INFECTIONS OF THE ARMS, LEGS, OR HANDS

Take a high pressure cold shower (see Hydrotherapy). This will increase circulation to the area and help reduce the inflammation.

- Aromatherapy - Inhale or apply near area of infection any one of the following oils: borneo, camphor, eucalyptus, garlic, lavender, lemon, onion, pine, thyme or clove.

## INFLUENZA (SEE ENTRY ON RESPIRATORY DISORDERS).

- Supplementation - Supplements that you can use to help reduce the effects of this condition include vitamin A, B complex, $B_1$, $B_2$, $B_6$, C, niacin and pantothenic acid.

- Tissue Salts - A combination of the following may be of help: - Take Nat. Sulph 6X.
- Aromatherapy - Inhale the aromatic oils of cinnamon, fennel and garlic to prevent influenza. Other effective aromatic oils include garlic, pine needles, thyme, hyssop, lavender, niaouli, onion, peppermint, rosemary, and sage.

## INSECT BITES AND STINGS

Placing commercial meat tenderizer on the area of the sting will reduce the inflammation. Apple cider vinegar applied topically also helps.

- Aromatherapy - Inhale the aromatic oils of basil, cinnamon, garlic, lavender, lemon, onion, sage, savory or thyme.

## IRRITABLE BOWEL SYNDROME (IBS)

IBS consists of many different conditions which are placed under this general heading. No matter what the symptoms are the following may be of help: recommendations should be applied:

- Avoid all coffee, tea, alcohol and tobacco.
- Avoid milk and milk products. Many people who are constipated or who suffer from Irritable Bowel Syndrome are sensitive to milk sugar. Milk sugar sensitivity is known as lactose intolerance. When milk is eliminated from the diet many of the symptoms of I.B.S. may disappear.

A number of healing juices are effective for IBS symptoms:

| | | |
|---|---|---|
| Spinach | Cucumber | Beet |
| Watercress | Celery | Tomato |
| Carrot | Cabbage | |

IBS symptoms will sometimes appear as constipation. When this happens experts recommend the following course of action

1. Add l tablespoon of raw millers bran to a combination of apple, blueberry, and lemon juices. Eat whole grain cereal. Rice and oat bran are excellent sources of fiber. If you use wheat bran take it with plenty of fluid. Bran will help loosen your stools without irritating the bowels the way laxatives may.

2. Some people who have sluggish bowels may have a sensitivity to wheat. If so, try switching to a wheat free bread. Use barley, kasha, or corn and corn bran as a supplementary fiber source.

3. Other excellent sources of fiber include cabbage, dried fruit, apples, prunes, carrots, peas, spinach, bananas, pears, beets, corn and dried beans.

4. Increase your intake of sprouted seeds, such as alfalfa, mung beans, and sunflower.

5. Add a tablespoon of olive oil daily to your regular diet. This will help to increase normal intestinal functioning in a gentle way.

IBS symptoms will sometimes appear as diarrhea. When this happens experts recommend the following course of action

1. Drink plenty of water with a little honey and acidophilus added.

2. Juicing - Do not use juices in the acute phase of diarrhea. Take juices only as healing begins to take place. Then drink a combination of carrot, alfalfa, sprout, and beet juice to which you've added a trace-mineral supplement. The mineral supplement is available in a health food store and is recommended to replace those minerals lost from diarrhea.

3. Once the loose stools have subsided emphasize high fiber foods including whole grains, beans, fresh fruits and vegetables.

## JAUNDICE

This is a symptom that may occur with a variety of diseases, including hepatitis. See a holistic physician before you self-treat. For acute conditions, go on a juice fast for one to two weeks.

- Use a coffee enema every two days.
- Place cabbage leaf compresses over the liver area.
- Several times a day, drink Barley water (1 cup of barley boiled in 6 pints of water and simmered for three hours).

• Supplementation - Supplements that you can use to help reduce the effects of this condition include vitamin A, B[6], C,D, E, EFA, pantothenic acid, C (3-5 grams daily). Other

recommended supplements include calcium, lecithin, magnesium, phosphorous, and brewers yeast.
- Herbs - Drink teas or extracts of Irish moss, dandelion,
  horsetail, gentian, parsley, fennel or centaury,
- Aromatherapy - Inhale the aromatic oils of geranium,
  lemon, rosemary and thyme.

## LACTATION (TO STIMULATE)

- Aromatherapy - Inhale the aromatic oils aniseed, caraway,
  fennel.

## LACTATION (TO DRY UP)

- Aromatherapy - Inhale the aromatic oils sage, peppermint.

## LACTOSE INTOLERANCE

Deficiency of lactase enzyme results in the inefficient digestion of
lactose (milk sugar), a condition called lactose intolerance.
Acidophilus produces lactase enzyme which helps digest lactose.

## LARYNGITIS

Marion Brand Throat Lozenges are used by many opera singers for this
problem. It does contain refined sugar which is unfortunate but the
singers I know swear by the product (available at most pharmacies).

- Aromatherapy - Inhale the aromatic oils lemon, cypress,
  thyme, cajuput, sage.

- Hydrotherapy - Wrap a moist warm cloth around your neck.
  Place a dry cloth over it.

## LEAD TOXICITY -

1. In children - Many holistic medical doctors recommend high
   dosage intravenous supplementation of Vit. C (30-40 grams)
   with calcium at frequent intervals. Many articles and studies
   have been published about Vit. C and lead poisoning.
2. Lead may be a contributing factor to hypertension.

3. Lead toxicity

- Supplementation - Supplements that you can use to help reduce the effects of this condition include Calcium, Vitamin A, $B_1$, C, lecithin and algin.
- Nutrition - Use plenty of legumes and beans. The fiber in these foods helps reduce toxic metal levels in the body.

## LICE

- Aromatherapy - Inhale the aromatic oils lavender, eucalyptus, mustard, terebinth, thyme.

## LICHEN PLANUS

- Supplementation - Vitamins that you can use to help reduce the effects of this condition include $B_1$, $B_6$, C.

## LIVER PROBLEMS

- Juice Therapy - For a healthy liver, try these recommendations:
- Drink Juice Therapy Formula #18 or #25 (twice daily)
- Squeeze ten lemons in two quarts of water and drink a glass of the mixture every two hours. Sweeten the lemon water with or maple syrup to taste.
- Juice Therapy -Among the many combinations to help heal the liver the following are most popular:
- For an enlarged liver, drink papaya juice.
- Grape juice is a very good healing juice for general liver problems.
- Drink a combination of carrot, beet, and dandelion juices.
- To promote bile activity, add lemon juice to water and drink this mixture in the morning.

## LOW BODY TEMPERATURE

- Aromatherapy - Inhaling certain aromatic oils stimulate circulation and the resulting warmth will increase body temperature if it is low. Among the most important benzoin, camphor, cinnamon, juniper, sage and thyme.

## LUPUS ERYTHEMATOSUS

- Supplementation - Supplements you can use to help reduce the effects of this condition are vitamin $B_1$, $B_6$, C, A, and the mineral manganese. Vitamin E taken orally and topically has been found to reduce the reddish, scaly blotches of the cutaneous (discoid) form of the disease. (*Cutis*, January 1979) 800-1600 IU of vitamin E seems to be the most effective dosage.

   - Externally applied PABA cream may also be of value.

- Juice Therapy - Try a glass of carrot juice in the morning and in the evening.
- Aromatherapy - Inhale oil of Clove. Avoid sunbathing.

## LUPUS VULGARIS

Vitamins you can use to help reduce the effects of this condition are $B_1$, $B_6$, C. D, C.

## MALE SEXUAL AND REPRODUCTIVE PROBLEMS

- Juice Therapy - Try therapy Formula #6 . Two very popular juice combinations are: (1) Combine equal parts carrot and spinach juices; and (2) Mix carrot, asparagus, and lettuce juices.

## MEASLES

The fever associated with this condition increases the body's need for vitamin A and C. Caloric requirements are also increased.

- Juice Therapy - Try a glass of Carrot/Beet juice. Increased fluid intake of all types is important to reducing the symptoms of measles. It is best to eat frequent small meals rather than a few large ones.

## MENOPAUSE

- Juice Therapy - Formulas #2 and #6 are very helpful. Also, try drinking a glass of ice water at the first sign of symptoms.

## MENINGITIS

This condition requires prompt medical attention. There is an increased need for vitamin A and C due to the high fever associated with this condition.

## MOTION SICKNESS

This condition generally starts in the gastrointestinal tract and the central nervous system.

- Herbs - Studies indicate that ginger root affects both systems in such a way as to prevent nausea and vomiting. Other herbs for reducing motion sickness include red raspberry leaves, hyssop, meadow sweet, peppermint leaves.

## MULTIPLE SCLEROSIS

Cold climates seem to aggravate the symptoms.

- Nutrition - Though there is no cure for this condition there have been some benefits associated with certain dietary approaches. These include:
- Increase intake of linoleic acid (found in sunflower seed oil).
- Increased intake of unsaturated fats such as wheat germ oil, pumpkin seed or sunflower seed oil.
- Increase intake of Vitamin E Carrot/celery juice (equal parts).

Dietary Suggestions

- The MacDougall Diet has been reported to produce some results if adhered to over a period of time (even years). This is a gluten free diet that also limits saturated fats, alcoholic beverages, refined sugars and processed foods.

- Edgar Cayce- Massage the entire body with Cayce's Arthritis Massage Formula. Massage seems to reduce the symptoms in many MS patients..

- Supplementation - Supplementation you can use to help reduce the effects of this condition include vitamin $B_1$, $B_6$, $B_{12}$, C, E, niacin, and pantothenic acid. Other recommended nutrients include choline, lecithin, EFA, and the minerals manganese, calcium and magnesium. Supplementation with the amino acid Taurine has been found to reduce leg cramping and other muscular symptoms.

- Hyperbaric Oxygen Therapy - According to a medical report in the journal *Medical Month* (December 1983, p. 67) this approach has been shown in a controlled research study to improve bladder control, mobility, balance and stamina in M.S. patients. A double blind study found that patients breathing 90% oxygen had symptom remissions far more often that others getting 10% oxygen in a chamber. (New England Journal of Medicine, Jan 27, 1983).

## MUSCULAR DYSTROPHY

- Supplementation - Some preliminary reports indicate that Glutamic acid may be of some value in treating this disorder. The amino acid Glycine has been useful in maintenance of degenerative muscular diseases including Muscular Dystrophy.

- Nutrition - In the early stage of the disease increased protein intake may help slow down muscular wasting. Use more grain and bean combinations and fermented dairy products.

## MUSCULOSKELETAL PROBLEMS

- Juice Therapy - Try juice therapy Formula #16 to strengthen your bone structure.

## NAIL PROBLEMS (BRITTLE, THINNING, DRYING, EXCESSIVE RIDGING)

- Supplementation - Supplements you can use to help reduce the effects of this condition are vitamin $B_1$, $B_6$, C, and folic acid. Other recommended supplements include calcium, iron, brewer's yeast, silica, Evening Primrose Oil, zinc, and Betaine HCL.

- Aromatherapy - Inhale the aromatic oil lemon.
- Juice Therapy therapy - Use a combination of cucumber, parsnip and green pepper. Juice therapy formula #11 will give you the natural silica to strengthen brittle nails.
- Tissue salt - Brittle nails respond to combination of Kali Sulph., Nat. Mur., Silicea.
- Herbs - Use Horsetail as a tea, tablet or extract.

## NERVOUS DISORDERS (GENERAL)

This condition actually includes hundreds of disorders and abnormal situations rather then one specific disorder.

- Supplementation - Supplements you can use to help reduce the effects of this condition are the B Vitamins. B Complex deficiencies are often a cause or part of a rehabilitation program for illness of this type.
- Herbs - Drink teas made from these herbs ginger, peppermint, spearmint.
- Supplementation - Supplements you can use to help reduce the effects of this condition are papain and bromelain.
- Juice Therapy - Formula #2 is healing to the nervous system.

- Massage the body with the Edgar Cayce recommended arthritis massage formula. It may be of value in a wide range of nervous disorders.

## NEURITIS

- Supplementation - Supplements you can use to help reduce the effects of this condition are vitamin $B_1$, $B_6$, C, and the rest of the vitamin B complex, including, $B_2$, $B_6$, $B_{12}$, niacin, and pantothenic acid. Other recommended supplements include magnesium, silica, and brewer's yeast.
- Juice Therapy - try these juices: carrot, beet, apple, pineapple or any citrus juices.

## NIGHT BLINDNESS

- Supplementation - Vitamin A is a supplement you can use to help reduce the effects of this condition. If Vitamin A does not produce the desired result then use the B complex, especially $B_1$, $B_2$, and Niacin. The mineral zinc is also of value in this condition.

## NOSEBLEEDS

- Supplementation -Supplements you can use to help reduce the effects of this condition are vitamin K and Bioflavonoids. Your doctor may perform a test called Prothrombin Time (protime for short) to determine if low levels of vitamin K are the cause of your condition. Full healing may take up to six weeks. Chlorophyll is also valuable. The best way to get chlorophyll is to increase your intake of green leafy vegetables.
- Aromatherapy - Inhale the aromatic oils of lemon, terebinth.

## OBESITY

Unless you are on a supervised juice therapy program, you should avoid most fruit and vegetables juices while you are following a weight-loss program. Many dieters drink large quantities of juices because they consider juices lower in calories. However, many juices may actually be higher in calories; at the same time, juices do not have the benefit of fiber.

- Juice Therapy formula that you will find helpful: Add to a 16-ounce glass of combined carrot, beet, and apple juices one teaspoon of bee pollen. This formula will help support your glandular function.

If you are too overweight, your chances of developing some chronic disorders are increased. Obesity is associated with high blood pressure, increased levels of blood fats (triglycerides) and cholesterol, and the most common type of diabetes. All of these, in turn, are associated with increased risks of heart attacks and strokes. Thus, you should try to maintain your "ideal" weight.

It is not well understood why some people can eat much more

than others and still maintain normal weight. However, one thing is certain: to lose weight, you must take in fewer calories than you burn. This means that you must either select foods containing fewer calories or you must increase your activity — or both.

If you need to lose weight, do so gradually. A steady loss of 1 to 2 pounds a week — until you reach your goal — is relatively safe and more likely to be maintained. Long-term success depends upon acquiring new and better habits of eating and exercise.

Avoid crash diets that are severely restricted in the variety of foods they allow. Diets containing fewer than 800 calories may be hazardous to your health. Some people have developed kidney stones, disturbing psychological changes, and other complications while following such diets. A few people have died suddenly.

## OSTEOMALACIA

- Supplementation - Supplements you can use to help reduce the effects of this condition include vitamin D, and Betaine HCL for older patients. Sunshine is an important healer as well.

## OSTEOPOROSIS

Osteoporosis is becoming a major cause of injury, particularly among postmenopausal women. Lack of dietary calcium is often a factor in the disease, and lactic bacteria has been shown to favorably affect calcium intake and absorption.

- Nutrition - To increase your calcium increase your intake of broccilli, kale, sea vegetables and dairy products. Yogurt, kefir, buttermilk, and other cultured dairy products are best.

Avoid eating excessive amounts of protein, especially beef and other meats. Excessive protein results in a loss of calcium. Calcium may be lost when sulfur containing amino acids are metabolized. Meat is high in sulfur-containing amino acids and would contribute to this loss of calcium.

Not surprisingly, lacto and lacto-ovo vegetarians in their 70's and 80's generally have a greater bone mass and a lower incidence of osteoporosis than meat eaters in their 60's.

Also, use high-mineral foods, which include:

| | |
|---|---|
| Sea vegetables | Green vegetables |
| Whole grains | Strawberries, blueberries & |
| Cabbage Raspberries | Raw, unsalted nuts and seeds |

Because calcium increases bone density, be sure to include calcium lactate or calcium carbonate in your daily diet. Studies show that calcium can even increase bone density in the elderly.


## PAIN

- Herbs - willow bark and leaves

To increase your threshold for pain, follow a diet high in carbohydrates, low in fats, and low in proteins. Try TENS Therapy.

- Supplementation - The amino acid DL-Phenylalanine has been found to be helpful for the reduction of arthritis pain (This amino acid should be avoided if you suffer from a condition called PKU. Check with your physician).
- Nutrition - Reduce your corn intake. Studies show that people who followed corn-rich diets had a lower tolerance for pain, perhaps because corn is low in L-Tryptophan.

Include these Tryptophan-rich foods in your diet:

| | |
|---|---|
| Soybeans and soy proteins | Yogurt |
| Cottage cheese | Brown rice |
| Mixed nuts | Raw, unsalted pumpkin & |
| Baked beans | sesame seeds |
| Lentils | Avocados |
| Bananas | Pineapples |
| Green leafy vegetables | |

Include these Phenylalanine-rich foods in your diet: nuts soybeans, and other beans.

Except for protein foods listed above, avoid concentrated proteins like meat, fish, eggs, or poultry in a pain-control program. These foods may reduce Tryptophan levels and serotonin levels. Instead , eat complex carbohydrates

## PANCREATITIS

- Juice Therapy - The powdered juice of young-green-barley plants may be of help. It is available in the United States as Green Magma.

## PARASITES (INTESTINAL)

There are many different folk remedies for the destruction of intestinal parasites. Garlic juice, and raw unsalted pumpkin seeds are among the most popular.

## PARKINSONS DISEASE

According to recent studies done at Yale University School of medicine when protein was limited to seven grams a day and was consumed at dinner, it produced a marked relief in several disabled subjects, yet did not result in protein deficiency as measured by levels of albumin, a protein carried in the blood. Beginning a regime of this type should be done under a physicians supervision.

Other health building approaches for those suffering from this condition include:

- Juice Therapy - Try a combination of Carrot/celery juice (equal parts).
- Use the vitamin B complex to support nerve tissue.
- Use a High fiber diet to reduce constipation.
- Increase fluid intake to offset the drug side effects of reduced intestinal secretions.

- Supplementation - you can use to help reduce the effects of this condition include vitamin $B_6$, $B_2$, C, and E as well as glutamic acid, lecithin, magnesium., calcium.
- Herbs - Ginseng, damiana, cayenne are all herbs that can be taken in capsule form.

## PELLEGRA

- Supplementation - Supplements you can use to help reduce the effects of this condition include all of the B vitamins especially $B_1$, $B_2$, and niacin.

## PERSPIRATION (EXCESSIVE)

- Herbs - Apply any of the following teas or liquids to the skin; apple cider vinegar, pekoe tea, witch hazel, white oak bark. These are astringents which may cause the sweat ducts to close, thus preventing perspiration from reaching the surface of the skin.

## PERICARDITIS

- Aromatherapy - Inhale the aromatic oil of onion.

## PHARYNGITIS

- Aromatherapy - Inhale the aromatic oil of Cajuput.

## PHLEBITIS

- Supplementation - Vitamins you can use to help reduce the effects of this condition include vitamin B complex, C, E, niacin, and pantothenic acid.

- Herbs - Butchers broom can be used as an herb tea or in extract form. (see any recommendations for improving circulation).

- Aromatherapy - Inhale the aromatic oil of Lemon.

## POISON IVY

As soon as you make contact with poison Ivy rub the crushed leaves of the Jewel Weed or plantain plant on the affected area to reduce itching. If that isn't possible the next best thing is to wash the rash with buttermilk to dry it up.

Other approaches include:

- Nutrition and herb Suggestions - You can coat or wash the affected areas with any of the following; aloe vera gel, vitamin E oil, a baking soda poultice. 2,000 mg.
- Supplementation - 2,000 mg. of vitamin C should be taken daily to eccelerate the healing.

• Miscellaneous

- Wash area with an organic solvent such as rubbing alcohol, then, wash the area liberally with plain cold water
- Avoid using soap since this removes the protective oils from the skin.
- Avoid using a wash cloth since this can pick up resins and reinfect you.
- Wash all clothing that may have made contact with the plant since resins can remain potent for as long as a year.

## POISON OAK

Wash the rash with buttermilk to dry up the inflammation.

## POLYCYTHEMIA

• Juice Therapy - Fast with an emphasis on red grape, black current and beet juice.

## RADIOACTIVE CONTAMINATION

• Supplementation - To reduce the risk of contamination use kelp tablets and other seaweeds, red miso, liquid iodine, potassium, algin based supplements, vitamin E, selenium and any other of the antioxidants available.

## RECTAL ITCH

• Folk Remedies - There are a number of popular remedies for solving this problem. Among them are:

- rubbing the anal opening with an ice cube
- A hot sitz bath (just fill the tub high enough so that the water only covers the lower part of your body. After bath apply any of the following with absorbent cotton; lemon juice, apple cider vinegar, wheat germ oil.

## RESPIRATORY DISORDERS

• Nutrition - In respiratory disorders, try to avoid the foods that many asthmatics are particularly sensitive to:

| | |
|---|---|
| Milk | Chocolate |
| Orange Juice | Butter |
| Fish | Peanut Butter |
| Nuts | |

• Supplementation - Many supplements can be especially
  helpful in avoiding and relieving respiratory disorders:

- Vitamin $B_6$ -In a Columbia University study, a daily dose
  of 100 milligrams of vitamin $B_6$ produced fewer and less
  severe asthma attacks and at the same time reduced short-
  ness of breath and other symptoms. But for best results,
  many nutritionists recommend taking 200 milligrams daily,
  especially for asthmatic children.
- Vitamin C - Because Vitamin C expands the air passages,
  it is especially effective in relieving the effects of cold and
  asthma symptoms. Furthermore, vitamin C has been found
  to reduce the number and severity of asthma attacks in
  asthmatics as well as the severity of bronchospasms.

• Juice Therapy - Formula #5 may help bring relief from
  any respiratory disorder—especially asthma, bronchitis,
  pneumonia, and emphysema. Also valuable for respiratory disorders is a combination of celery juice and parsnip
  juice.

For emphysema, add four ounces of raw potato juice to Juice
Therapy Formula #12.


### RESTLESS LEG SYNDROME

Causes of this condition may include anemia, excessive use of caffeine, previous excess exposure to cold temperatures and certain
drugs and general nutritional deficiencies.

• Supplementation - Supplements that you can use to help
  reduce the effects of this condition include vitamin E, calcium and cayenne pepper (taken in capsule form).

## RETROLENTAL FIBROPLASIA (RLF)

- Supplementation - Some studies have indicated that vitamin E may reduce the severity of this condition.

## REYES SYNDROME

This rare but serious illness often afflicts children who have been given aspirin for chicken pox or flu symptoms. If you believe your child has one of these conditions do not give them aspirin. Speak with a physician about this matter.

## RHINITIS

Rest and increased fluid intake are key to healing from this condition.

- Supplementation - Vitamin A can help reduce the effects of this condition.
- Aromatherapy - Inhale the aromatic oils of basil, niaouli, thyme.

## RICKETS

- Supplementation - You can help reduce the effects of this condition by including vitamin D, and the minerals calcium and/or phosphorous in your diet.

## RINGWORM

Apply apple cider vinegar to the affected area several times daily. You may also wish to rub the area with powdered borax, chestnut oil or castor oil.

## ROUNDWORM, (ASCARIS)

- Aromatherapy - Inhale the aromatic oils of eucalyptus, thyme, lavender, chamomile.

## SCABIES

- Aromatherapy - A drop of the essence of lavender, lemon, rosemary, orange flower, cloves, cinnamon, mustard or thyme will kill the scabies mite. Tea Tree Oil is also very effective.

## SCARS

- Edgar Cayce recommends a formula containing lanolin, olive oil, camphor and peanut oil to reduce external scars.

## SCLERODERMA

Relaxation training may be helpful in relieving stress, which can often aggravate symptoms of this condition. Physical therapy and an exercise program alternated with periods of rest is highly recommended.

## SCROFULOSIS

- Aromatherapy - Inhale the aromatic oils of lavender, onion, sage.

## SCURVY

- Nutrition - This condition is a result of a vitamin C deficiency. Vitamin C or foods rich in this vitamin will reduce the effects of this condition. You should also increase your intake of bioflavanoids and increase your intake of citrus fruits, green peppers, and onions.
- Aromatherapy - Inhale the aromatic oils of ginger, lemon, onion.

## SENSORY DISORDERS (LOSS OF TASTE AND SMELL)

- Supplementation - Zinc deficiency is a common cause of this condition. Zinc lozenges should be taken under the tongue for best absorption. They are available in most health food stores.

## SHINGLES

- Supplementation - Vitamin E should be applied directly to the lesions. Vitamin E should also be taken orally in doses up to 1600 IU daily.

- Vitamin C injections have been shown to reduce the pain and dry up lesions.

- Vitamin A & C will help to increase healing of the skin lesions.
- A physician can give you intramuscular injections of thiamine hydrochloride and vitamin $B_{12}$.
- Other supplements you can use to help reduce the effects of this condition include rutin, the vitamin B complex, calcium, lecithin, EFA (Essential Fatty Acids.)
- Apple cider vinegar can be applied topically, several times a week.
- Hot baths have also been shown to be of help to some people.

- Aromatherapy - Inhale the aromatic oils of cajuput, geranium, citral.

## SHOCK

- Aromatherapy - Inhale the aromatic oils of camphor melissa and niaouli.

## SICKLE CELL ANEMIA

- Supplementation - Supplements that you can use to help reduce the effects of this condition include vitamin $B_6$, E and the mineral zinc. Vitamin $B_6$ has been found to reduce some of the symptoms of this condition that affects African-Americans. Zinc supplementation can help patient growth return to normal. The zinc should be taken between meals to aid in its absorption. Studies have shown that vitamin E can reduce irreversibly sickled cells by limiting the effect of the oxidation process that can contribute to this condition. A low sodium diet limits the number and severity of crises experienced by those stricken.

## SINUSITIS

- Juice Therapy - For mucus congestion, try Juice Therapy Formula #5, and one hour later follow it up by drinking a combination of 12 ounces of carrot juice and 4 ounces of radish juice.

- Horseradish, one of the ingredients in Juice Therapy

Formula #5, dissolves mucus. The radish juice then cleanses the body of this dissolved mucus, according to N.W. Walker, the pioneer of juice therapy.

## SKIN DISORDERS

- Juice Therapy - Try juice therapy Formula #3. Another great juice formula is a combination of green pepper juice and raw potato juice (half-and-half). This formula should not be used if you have arthritis. This is because nightshade plants like peppers and potatoes can aggravate the symptoms of this condition. Another popular approach is to drink 16 ounces of carrot juice each day. Other popular juice therapies for specific skin disorders include:
- For Boils - Try Juice Therapy Formulas #14, #17, and 20.
- For Acne - Mix the juice of carrots, lettuce, and spinach in equal parts. Some food allergies may contribute to acne, especially allergies to dairy products and wheat.
- Nutrition - To follow a nutrition program that will help promote healthy skin and treat any skin disorders, be sure to avoid:

| Yeast | Alcohol | Strong spices |
|---|---|---|
| Wheat products | Black teas | Very hot foods & beverages |
| Refined sugar | Coffee | Cow's milk |

Cow's milk is a common allergen for people with skin problems. Although not everyone with a skin problem is allergic to cow's milk, many people who replace cow's milk with goat's milk or soy milk get rid of their rashes or dermatitis symptoms.

Be sure to include essential fatty acids in your diet. Studies show that EFAs are a major factor in healing skin disorders. To obtain EFAs, add a few tablespoons of sesame oil, safflower oil, or sunflower oil daily either to your salad or to the foods you cook. Other good sources of EFA's are raw, unsalted nuts and seeds.

Specifics:

**Bedsores** - A protein deficiency can contribute to or aggravate bedsores or ulcers. If your protein intake is not adequate, supplement your diet with soy or milk based protein powders. These are available at most health food stores..

**Burns** - Extreme burns may require intravenous feeding and hospitalization. If you are an average-size person, increase your caloric intake to 5,000 or 6,000 calories a day and your protein intake to 200 grams a day. Also eat many small meals rather than a few large meals.

**Eczema** - Protein deficiencies have also been found to cause eczema. Increase your intake of fermented milk products and grain and bean combinations.

**Psoriasis** - The cause of psoriasis is not known, but many patients see improvement in their conditions when they start a gluten-free diet and eliminate acidic foods, such as coffee, pineapples, tomatoes, soda, corn, nuts, and milk. An increased intake of animal protein may aggravate psoriasis.

## SLEEP DISORDERS

- Juice Therapy - For general sleep disorders, drink the juice of eight to ten celery stalks each day. Celery juice is an excellent source of magnesium, sodium, and iron.

Also try a combination of carrot and celery juice.

To promote a healthy sleeping pattern, follow this basic nutritional advice:

- Avoid alcohol and coffee, as well as all other caffeinated beverages.
- Eat your meals at the same time each day.
- Avoid eating a large meal in the evening, and always avoid eating for at least 2 hours before you go to bed.
- At your evening meal, increase your carbohydrate intake and decrease your protein intake.
- Eating high-carbohydrate foods with some fats (such as vegetable oils) may increase your level of serotonin, which helps you sleep easier.
- Be sure to eat plenty of foods rich in tryptophan such as cheddar cheese, cottage cheese, whole milk, and skim milk
- Losing weight may be helpful if you suffer from sleep apnea.

## SMOKING (CESSATION)

Studies indicate that both underweight and highly obese smokers exhibited death rates 10% higher than ideal weight smokers. A natural way to quit smoking is to chew small pieces of dried calamus root (no more than 4 per day). Chewing this herb will give you a strong aversion toward cigarettes.

- Supplementation -To reduce the effects of tar and nicotine on your body it is wise to take take vitamins A, C, E, $B_6$, $B_{12}$, and the mineral calcium.

## SNEEZING

The causes of persistent sneezing may include polyps in the nose, allergies and emotional factors. Avoid blocking the explosive phase since this can result in a dangerous increase of blood pressure in the head. If the sneezing does not stop, deliberately increasing it may wear out the reflex temporarily and halt the attack. When the sneezing is the result of stimulation of the involuntary nervous system use massage by kneading the neck and the abdomen to stop the attack.

## SORE THROAT

- Supplementation - Vitamins and supplements that you can use to help reduce the effects of this condition include vitamin A, C & D as well as the minerals calcium, magnesium, and zinc.
- Herbs - recommended herbs include slippery elm bark lozenges, golden seal extract, and a tea made from plantain leaves, and ginger.
- Aromatherapy - Inhale the aromatic oils of geranium, ginger, lemon, sage, thyme.

## SPITTING OF BLOOD

- Herbs - Whether the blood comes from the lungs or the kidneys, horsetail or blood wort tea has used by European herbalists effectively. See a holistic physician if the bleeding does not stop.

## SLIPPED DISC

- Supplementation - Vitamin C can help reduce the effects of this condition.

## STOMATITIS

- Supplementation - A supplement you can use to help reduce the effects of this condition is barley juice powder (Green Magma Brand).

- Aromatherapy - Inhale the aromatic oils of geranium, lemon, sage.

## STY (ON THE EYE)

Place a compress of cold water on the sty. A popular folk remedy for the relief of a sty is to place a pot cheese compress on the affected eye.

- Tissue salt - Try Silicia. If the sty is inflamed alternate silicea with Ferr. Phos.

## SWEATING (PROFUSE)

- Aromatherapy - Inhale the aromatic oils of pine, cypress.
- Supplementation - Zinc lozenges can help reduce the effects of this condition.

## SWELLING OF THE FEET

- Hydrotherapy - Sponge the entire body with warm water. Soak the feet in a pail of warm water with a few table spoons of vinegar added. A physician should be sought out to determine if any heart or kidney problems are causing the swelling.

## TACHYCARDIA (RAPID HEARTBEAT)

This may not necessarily be a disorder but rather a normal reaction to stress. To reduce this problem put your face in a basin of very cool water (Lancet, Jan. 4, 1975). Check with your physician before attempting this technique since it is contraindicated for certain types of Tachycardia. Avoid the use of caffeine, tobacco products and alcohol.

- Supplementation - Minerals that help reduce the effects of this condition include magnesium and potassium.

- Aromatherapy - Inhale the aromatic oils of Ylang-ylang, garlic.

## TAPEWORM

- Aromatherapy - Inhale the aromatic oils of terebinth, thyme, garlic.

## TARDIVE DYSKINESIA

- Supplementation - Vitamins and supplements that you can use to help reduce the effects of this condition include Choline, lecithin, vitamins C, E, B6 and niacin.
- Herbs - Chewing Betel Nut will help to reduce the symptoms associated with this condition. (Betel Nuts should be used in moderation. They can found in East Indian supply stores).

## TEETHING IN CHILDREN

- Tissue Salt - A combination of the following may be of help; Calcarea Phos. 6X, Kali. Phos. Kali Sulph. 12X, Nat. Phos.

## TENNIS ELBOW

Spray the inflamed area with catalyst altered water (Also known as Willard's Water. This is found in many natural food stores)

## THRUSH

- Aromatherapy - Inhale the aromatic oils of geranium, lemon sage

## THYROID (UNDERACTIVE)

- Supplementation - Supplements that you can use to help reduce the effects of this condition include kelp, and vitamin C & E. It is also helpful to add a tablespoon of extra-virgin olive oil daily to your diet.

- Herbs - Use an extract of any of the following herbs: golden seal, bayberry, myrrh, and black cohosh.

Avoid "goitrogenic" foods (these are foods that can interfere with the formation of thyroid hormones by the thyroid gland.) Foods classified in this category include; Brussel sprouts, cabbage, cauliflower, kale, kohlrabi, rutabaga, turnips and soybeans and soy products such as tempeh and tofu.

## TINGLING IN THE FINGERS

- Supplementation - When tingling is associated with fatigue you should increase your intake of of vitamin $B_6$ since a deficiency of this nutrient can cause these symptoms.

## TINNITIS -

Causes may include allergies, alcohol, tobacco, cocaine, marijuana, caffeine but none of these has been clearly established. Some people believe that the symptoms of tinnitis, which include ringing in the ears can be controlled by stabilizing blood sugar. This can be done by using a whole foods diet spread out over six small meals and avoiding refined sugar, coffee, tea and alcohol.

## TONGUE (A BURNING SENSATION OF)

This may be caused by digestive problems, tobacco usage, emotional factors, condiments, mouth infections, jagged teeth. Cleansing the tongue with a soft toothbrush after eating may avoid irritation from tiny food particles that may become lodged in the tongue's many projections.

## TONSILLITIS

- Supplementation - Vitamins that you can use to help reduce the effects of this condition include folic acid and vitamin C.
- Tissue Salts - A combination of the following may be of help: Ferrum Phos, Kali Mur, Kali Phos. may be of help.
- Aromatherapy - Inhale the aromatic oils of geranium, lemon, ginger, sage, thyme.

## TUBERCULOSIS

- Nutrition -A vegetarian high protein diet is recommended.
- Supplementation - Supplementation that you can use to help reduce the effects of this condition include vitamin A, niacin, pantothenic acid, $B_6$, $B_{12}$, C, and D. Important minerals that should be taken are calcium, iron, and phosphorus.
- Aromatherapy - According to studies published in France the "essences of palmaros, cinnamon and cloves in particular were found to be active with regard to homogeneous cultures of the tuberculosis bacillus." Other healing oils included cajuput, eucalyptus, lemon, niaoli, origanum, pine, terebinth, and thyme.

## UREA (EXCESS IN BLOOD) AZOTAEMIA

- Aromatherapy - This condition responds to the aromatic oil of garlic.

## URETHRITIS

- Aromatherapy - Inhale the aromatic oils of cajuput, niaouli, terebinth.

## URINARY TRACT DISORDERS

- Nutrition - Diet and food can help in general disorders of the urinary tract, including kidney and bladder disorders.

The following recommendations should be of assistance:

- Follow a vegetarian diet that is low in protein and high in complex carbohydrates. Be sure to include plenty of steamed vegetables, raw fruits, salads, brown rice, and raw, certified goat's milk. You may also include yogurt, kefir, and other cultured-milk products.
- Eat frequent small meals.
- Avoid salt.
- Be sure to eat the foods that are considered most effective in healing urinary tract infections: parsley, watercress, celery, horseradish, asparagus, cucumber, potatoes, and watermelon.

## How Nutrition Can Help in Specific Conditions

Here are a number of recommendations for specific Urinary Tract disorders.

**Kidney Stones** - Your nutritional habits can help treat kidney stones:

- For Kidney Stones: Juice Therapy Formula #6.

- Contrary to old myths, cutting down on calcium intake over a long period of time does not reduce the potential for stone formation. Worse, the cutback in calcium may contribute to bone loss and osteoporosis.

- Using significant amounts of sugar and sugar products can increase your chances of calcium stone formation. If you have a history of forming stones, avoid foods high in oxalates including spinach, unhulled sesame seeds, chocolate, beets, pepper, rhubarb, tea, nuts, and figs.

- If you have calcium phosphate stones, avoid very concentrated alkaline foods, such as fruit juices and cola-based soft drinks. If the stone formation is associated with gout, be sure to drink a lot of fluids-three to four quarts daily-to reduce uric acid concentrations in your system.

- Increase your intake of high-fiber foods to reduce your chances of stone formation. People who produce large amounts of uric acid are susceptible to uric acid stones. Generally, these people consume large amounts of animal protein-meat, fish, and poultry and do not use many high-fiber foods.

- Lower your intake of high-fat foods. People with high-fat intakes have higher stone formation.

- Lower your intake of milk and milk products.

**Nephritis** - Reduce your protein intake.

• Juice Therapy - The first choice in juice therapy for urinary tract infections is unsweetened cranberry juice. In the early acute stages of kidney or bladder infection, avoid most fruit and vegetable juices, because they are too alkaline and may actually aggravate the condition.

• Juice Therapy - In addition, note these specific uses of juices

For **General Kidney Problems:** For **albuminuria, nephritis, and calculi of the kidney and bladder,** try these effective remedies:

- A combination of these juices: carrot, asparagus, and parsley.
- Juice Therapy Formula #2.
- Any one of these healing juices: watermelon, cucumber, or celery.
- Add watercress and garlic to carrot juice and drink this combination.
- For **Cystitis and Other Bladder Disorders:** Juice Therapy Formulas #6 and #17. Also drink unsweetened cranberry juice.
- As a Diuretic: Juice Therapy Formulas #4 and #5. When not combined with other juices, cucumber juice is one of the strongest and most effective natural diuretics.
- For **Urinary Tract Infections:** Drink cranberry juice for the first few days. Then as symptoms improve, start drinking carrot juice.

### The Role of Nutrition in Renal Insufficiency

In cases of renal insufficiency, the patient may be able to avoid a dialysis machine if he or she follows a special diet. The results of a recent research study indicate that "a low-protein, low-phosphorus diet supplemented with amino acids and keto acids can markedly influence the course of progressive chronic renal failure, as indicated by changes in the serum creatinine level." [Harvard Medical Area Focus, December 6, 1984, p. 1. *New England Journal of Medicine*, September 6, 1984, pp. 623-628.

For more information about this new nutritional approach to renal insufficiency, contact:

Harvard Medical Area News Office
25 Shattuck Street
Boston, MA 02115
(617) 732-1590

### VARICOSE VEINS (SWOLLEN ENLARGED VEINS)

People who work in occupations that require a large amount of standing seem more prone to this condition than those with sit-down jobs. Causes may include; poor diet, mineral deficiencies, inherited weakness in the structure of the vein, phlebitis, abdominal pressure form the stomach muscles (such as that caused by heavy lifting, coughing, straining, pregnancy, obesity and aging). This condition is common in the obese so the weight loss that comes through the application of the 30-Day Body Purification Program should be of great help.

Other approaches that may be of help include:

- avoiding tight clothing and crossing of the legs.
- Use support stockings.
- Stimulate your circulation by maintaining a consistent exercise program, especially if you must sit for long periods of time. Walking, running, bicycling or swimming are your best choices.
- Regular dry brush massage is also valuable for increasing circulation and promoting detoxification by means of the skin.
- Avoid standing in one place for an extended period of time.
- Women should avoid wearing tight girdles since this cuts off the circulation. If you insist on wearing a girdle never wear a girdle on the plane or any other place where you are going to be sitting for a long time. Support hose may be helpful in a mild condition.

• Aromatherapy - Inhale the aromatic oils of cajuput, niaouli, terebinth, cypress, garlic, lemon.
• Nutrition and supplementation - A high fiber diet helps create less pressure during bowel movements that can aggravate varicose veins.
• Supplementation -Vitamins and supplements that you can use to help reduce the effects of this condition include the vitamin B complex, C, E (800 - 2,400 iu daily if there is not hypertension), calcium, kelp, lecithin, and bioflavonoids.
• Juice Therapy - Try a combination of pineapple, grape, citrus, or carrot/spinach.
• Nutrition - A macrobiotic approach includes the elimination of "yin" (expansive) type foods. These include sugars, citrus fruit, cold liquids, fruit juice.

- Herbs - Use an extract of any of the following herbs: white oak bark, marigold, witch hazel, yarrow, mistletoe and butcher's broom.

## VERTIGO

- Aromatherapy - Inhale the aromatic oils of aniseed, basic, chamomile, caraway, lavender, peppermint, rosemary, sage, thyme.

## VITILIGO

- Supplementation - Supplements that you can use to help reduce the effects of this condition include PABA, pantothenic acid, and Betaine HCL.

## VOMITING

- Aromatherapy - Inhale the aromatic oils of aniseed, cajuput, fennel, peppermint.

## WARTS

- Aromatherapy - Inhale the aromatic oils of garlic, lemon, onion, thuja.

- Nutrition and Diet - Vitamin E oil applied to wart daily (800 i.u.) for a minimum of two months. A macrobiotic approach to treating plantar warts - reduce protein intake and apply grated raw eggplant or grated taro potato to the wart.

## WORMS

- Supplementation - Vitamins and supplements that you can use to help reduce the negative effects of this condition include vitamin A, B complex, ($B_1$, $B_2$, $B_6$, $B_{12}$, pantothenic acid,) D, K, EFA's and the minerals calcium iron, and potassium.

## WOUND HEALING

Increase protein intake.

- Supplementation - Vitamins and supplements that you can use to help increase wound healing include vitamin C, L-Ornithine, L- Arginine, DL-Carnitine. zinc, chromium (Federation proceedings, March 1, 1981). Natural vitamin E in cream or spray accelerates healing in hard to heal wounds. Propilis applied topically.
- Hydrotherapy - Chamomile compress to prevent infection of open wounds.
- Aromatherapy - Inhale the aromatic oils of cajuput, clove, eucalyptus, garlic, geranium, hyssop, juniper, lavender, niaouli, onion, rosemary, sage, savory, thyme.

If the wound is infected the focus should be on using wet dressings of the essence of chamomile and terebinth. Wet dressings promote the initial phase of healing faster than dry dressings.

## XANTHELASMA (FAT DEPOSITS ON THE EYELIDS) -

- Supplementation - A vitamin that you can use to help reduce the negative effects of this condition includes vitamin $B_{12}$ injections from your physician.

# PURIFICATION RECIPES

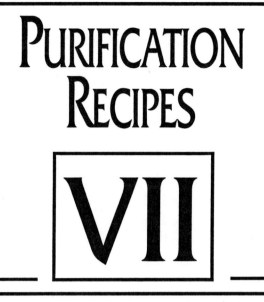

## VII

The following standard United States measurement guide should assist you in preparing our recommended recipes. You may adjust spice recommendations to suite your taste.

| U.S. Measurement Equivalents | |
| --- | --- |
| A pinch | = Less than 1/8 teaspoon |
| 1 teaspoon (tsp) | = 1/3 tablespoon |
| 1 tablespoon (T) | = 3 teaspoons |
| 2 tablespoons | = 1 fluid ounce |
| | |
| 8 fluid ounces | = 1 cup |
| 1 cup | = 16 tablespoons |
| 1 pint | = 2 cups |
| 16 fluid ounces | = 1 pint |
| 2 pints | = 1 quart |
| 4 quarts | = 1 gallon |
| 1/4 lb. butter | = 1/2 cup |

# COLD DISHES

### PINE NUT TABBOULEH

> 2/3 cup chopped unroasted pine nuts
> 1 cup bulghur (cracked wheat)
> 2/3 cup sliced green onions
> 1/2 cup lightly packed chopped parsley
> 2 tablespoons chopped mint leaves
> 1/2 cup raisins or dried currants
> 1/3 cup fresh squeezed lime or lemon juice
> 1/4 cup almond or olive oil
> 1/4 teaspoon pepper
> Romaine or Boston lettuce leaves

Measure bulghur into large bowl. Pour boiling distilled water over bulghur to just cover. Set aside about 30 minutes until water is completely absorbed. Add nuts and remaining ingredients except lettuce. Toss thoroughly. Cover and chill at least 2 hours. To serve, spread lettuce leaves on a serving plate and spoon wheat mixture onto the leaves. Makes 6 servings.

### MOCK-CHICKEN SALAD

> 2 or 3 most cups TVP (textured vegetable protein)
> 1/2 cup sliced fresh mushrooms
> 1/2 cup thinly sliced celery
> 2 tablespoons thinly sliced green onion
> 1/2 grated carrots
> 1/4 cup slivered almonds
> 2 tablespoons of eggless, low-fat Tofu-based mayonnaise
> (available at your health food store)

Combine the TVP, mushrooms, celery, green onion, carrots, and about half of the slivered almonds. Add the mayonnaise and toss until well mixed. Arrange on romaine and Boston lettuce leaves on a large salad plate or on individual plates. Garnish with remaining almonds. Makes 6 servings.

## HERBED TOFU PILAF

12 oz. Vegebase or vegetable powder mixed in distilled water
1 cup cracked wheat
1/2 teaspoon basil, crumbled
1/4 teaspoon mint flakes
1/2 teaspoon grated organically grown lemon rind
1/2 cup whole natural (unblanched) almonds
1 tablespoon almond or olive oil
1/2 cup sliced green onion
1/3 cup seedless raisins or currants
2 tablespoons chopped parsley
1 tablespoon lemon juice
1 cup diced tofu

Combine 12 oz. Vegebase and water with cracked wheat, basil, mint flakes, and lemon rind and heat to boiling. Cover, turn heat low, and cook 15 minutes. Meanwhile, chop almonds. When cracked wheat is cooked, add almonds, onion, raisins or (currants), parsley, and lemon juice; toss lightly to mix. Add tofu and heat a minute longer. Makes 3 servings.

## TEMPEH SALAD

2 cups cooked brown rice, chilled
1/2 cup thinly sliced celery
1/4 cup thinly sliced green onions with tops
1/4 cup sliced radishes
1 cup fresh bean sprouts or canned bean sprouts, drained
2 cups thinly slivered tempeh
1/2 cup slivered almonds, untoasted
1 tablespoon raw sesame seed,
1 tablespoon low sodium soy sauce
2 tablespoon apple cider vinegar
3 tablespoon almond or olive oil
Romaine or Boston lettuce
Fresh nectarine or peach slices

In a large bowl combine rice, celery, onions, radishes, bean sprouts, tempeh, and 1/4 cup of the almonds. Measure sesame seed, soy sauce, vinegar, and oil into small jar. Cover and shake well. Pour over rice mixture and toss thoroughly. Spoon into lettuce-lined bowl; chill. To serve, garnish with nectarine slices and remaining almonds. Makes 6 servings.

## TABBOULEH SALAD

> 1 cup bulghur wheat
>
> 2 cups boiling water
>
> 1/2 teaspoon sea salt
>
> 1 cup minced parsley
>
> 1/2 cup minced onion
>
> 1 or 2 ripe tomatoes, chopped (optional)
>
> 2 or 3 teaspoons dried mint or basil, or 1/4 cup fresh
>
> 1/4 cup olive oil
>
> Juice of 1 or 2 lemons

Pour boiling salted water over bulghur in medium-large salad bowl. Let sit for 10-15 minutes to absorb water, then stir to hasten cooling. Toss all other ingredients together with the soaked bulghur, adding garlic powder and/or pepper to taste. Let sit for 1/2 hour or more, if possible, to blend flavors. Serve on lettuce leaves as a salad, or stuff in Middle Eastern style pita bread for sandwiches. Makes about six servings.

### Variations:

Nearly any chopped or sliced vegetables go well in this flavorful salad: some possibilities are scallions, celery, chives, green pepper, cucumber, zucchini, avocado, mushrooms, sprouts, and spinach. A protein-rich salad can be made by adding cooked chickpeas of other beans, sunflower seeds, or chopped hard boiled eggs. The bulghur can also be cooked before using in salad: just add to boiling salted water and simmer for 30-40 minutes. Similar salads can be made with rice or pasta. With the many variations possible, you need never make the same salad twice!

# HOT LUNCH AND DINNER DISHES

Curried Rice
1/2 cups brown rice
4 cups water
1 teaspoon salt
2 tablespoons olive or canola oil
1 clove garlic, slivered
1/2 cup chopped onion
1/2 cup chopped green pepper
1/2 cup sunflower seeds
1/2 cup raisins
1/4 teaspoon curry powder

Wash rice; then add to 3 cups boiling salted water. Bring to a boil again, let boil for a minute, then reduce heat, and simmer, covered, for about 1 hour. Meanwhile, place frying pan on medium heat and add oil. When oil is hot, add onion, add garlic, and stir for a minute or two. Add green pepper, seeds, curry, and a pinch of salt and stir for another few minutes. Add raisins and 1 cup water, reduce heat, and simmer with lid ajar for 10 minutes or so, until liquid is half gone. Combine curry mixture with rice about 15 minutes before rice is done, mixing gently to keep rice fluffy. (Long-grain rice tends to cook fluffier than short or medium grain). Cook together without stirring until done, mix once lightly, and serve. Makes about 6 servings.

## CHILE BEAN BAKE

4 cups Mexican sauce
2/3 cup bulghur
1 1/2 cups cooked pinto beans

Mix all together. Pour into a large, oiled casserole and bake, covered, for 1 hour at 350° F. Mixture will be bubbly and fairly thick. Ladle into individual bowls and top each serving with shredded lettuce, chopped onion, thick yogurt, and shredded Monterey jack or dairy-free "soy" cheese. Serve with corn chips. Makes 6 servings.

## PARSLEY PASTA

> 1/2 pound whole wheat noodles or spaghetti
> 1 cup chopped parsley
> 1/4 teaspoon onion powder
> 1-2 tablespoon olive oil
> 1-2 teaspoon soy sauce

Cook pasta in boiling salted water for 10-12 minutes until done. Put parsley in large strainer, drain pasta by pouring directly onto parsley (this cooks it a bit). Toss with onion powder and oil and soy sauce, mixing well. Makes two to four servings.

### For Macaroni Salad:

Cook whole wheat elbow macaroni in boiling salted water. Meanwhile chop celery, green pepper, parsley, carrots, red onion, zucchini, and so on. Rinse macaroni thoroughly with cold water; then toss with vegetables and oil-and-vinegar dressing or soy (eggless) mayonnaise. Try cooking some tofu along with the macaroni, or using some cooked beans along with vegetables.

## CURRY BAKED TEMPEH

> 1-3/4 pounds of cubed tempeh
> 2/3 cup dairy low fat yogurt
> 1/2 teaspoon onion powder
> 1/8 teaspoon paprika
> 1/16 teaspoon curry powder
> 1 cup diced roasted almonds

Mix together low-fat yogurt, onion powder, paprika, and curry powder. Dip tempeh into yogurt-curry mixture. Roll tempeh pieces in almonds and arrange on flat baking pan. Bake in 350° F for about 25 minutes. Makes 4 servings.

## SPICY MUSHROOM-SAGE STUFFING

> 2 pounds fresh mushrooms,
> 3 tablespoons extra-virgin olive oil

4 large shallots, coarsely chopped

8 large garlic cloves, coarsely chopped

1 1/4 teaspoon thyme

1/2 cup coarsely chopped fresh sage

1 1/2 teaspoon freshly ground pepper

1 Tablespoon fresh squeezed lemon juice

1/2 teaspoon vegebase powder mixed in 2 oz. water

Wipe the mushrooms with a damp cloth and cut into 1/2-inch pieces; set aside.

In a large skillet or iron wok, heat the olive oil over moderately low heat. Add the shallots, garlic, and thyme and cook, stirring, until the shallots soften slightly, about 3 minutes. Increase the heat to moderately high and stir in the mushrooms. Cover and cook until the mushrooms soften, 5 to 6 minutes.

Add the sage, cayenne, and lemon juice and cook, stirring, until the mushrooms give off some of their liquid, 4 or 5 minutes. Season with salt and additional vegebase to taste. Transfer the stuffing to a large bowl and let cool to room temperature before using. (The stuffing can be made up to one day ahead.) Cover and refrigerate. Makes 4 servings

## MILLET-ONION SAUTE

1 medium yellow onion, chopped

1 tablespoons oil

2 cups cooked millet

Dash cayenne pepper

1/4 cup vegetable broth

2 tablespoons fresh chopped chives

In a large skillet, saute onion in hot oil until golden brown. Add millet, cayenne pepper, and vegetable broth. Stir to mix well. Heat thoroughly. Remove from heat and toss with chives. Makes 2 servings.

## BARLEY BURGERS

1 cup whole barley, blenderized for about 30 seconds at high speed (or medium pealed barley)

2 1/2 cups water

1 Tablespoon garlic powder (or 1 clove fresh garlic)

1 large onion, diced

1/2 cup chopped parsley (a handful)

1 Tablespoon canola oil

1/2 cup filberts (or other nuts)

1/2 teaspoon dried basil

1/2 teaspoon thyme

1/4 teaspoon oregano

Put garlic and barley in water. Boil about 10 minutes; set aside. Saute onion and parsley (or the parsley can be added later) with kelp and oil till tender, not soft.

When all the water has been absorbed by the barley grits, add the onion and all the other ingredients. Mix well. Allow to cool at least 30 minutes before forming burgers. Bake at 350° F for 40-45 minutes, turning once after about 20 minutes. Makes about 10-12 burgers.

## SOY BURGERS

1 large onion, minced

1 tablespoon oil

2 1/4 cups water

1 cup soy grits or granules

2 teaspoon kelp

2 tablespoons of Vegebase

1 teaspoon thyme

3 bay leaves

1/2 cup chopped parsley or 2 tablespoons dried

1/2 cup soy or other whole flour

1/2 cup dry whole wheat breadcrumbs or

1 cup soft whole wheat crumbs

Saute onion with oil in a small covered saucepan. If onion begins to burn, add 1 or 2 tablespoons water.

Add soy grits to boiling water. Add herbs, except fresh parsley if used. Boil gently about 10 minutes. Set aside. When water is absorbed — about 20 minutes — add onions and other remaining ingredients. (If water has not been absorbed, bring to a boil for another few minutes). Mix well. Form patties; place on oiled cookie sheet and bake at 350° F. for about 45 minutes, turning once after 20 minutes. Makes 12 medium burgers.

## PASTA VERDE

Cook the pasta ahead of time and refrigerate to save steps (and pots) when making your casserole. You have to cook the zucchini or it makes the casserole very watery.

> 1 1/2 cups cooked artichoke flour or whole wheat spaghetti or macaroni
> 2 tablespoons olive oil
> 1/3 cup mince scallions
> 1/2 clove garlic, minced
> 1 1/2 cups zucchini, thinly sliced
> 1/2 cup chopped parsley
> 1 teaspoon dried basil
> Freshly ground pepper
> Salt (optional)
> 1 1/2-2 cups Basic Mushroom Sauce

Cook the spaghetti or macaroni ahead of time and refrigerate. In a large skillet saute the scallions and the garlic in the oil for a few minutes. Do not brown. Add the zucchini and cook until the zucchini is tender-crisp and some of the water is cooked out of it. Add the parsley and seasonings and cook a few minutes more. Zucchini should be clear. Combine zucchini, spaghetti, and sauce and stir together well. Pour into an oiled casserole and bake at 350° F for 30-35 minutes. You can sprinkle some Parmesan cheese on top, if you like. Makes 2 to 4 servings.

## TOFU VEGETABLE CASSEROLE

This casserole is delicious and very easy to fix. If you can find fresh peas, steam them for a while first before you add the others. If using frozen peas, steam them last.

> 1 cup cubed raw potatoes, skins left on
> 1 cup fresh carrots, sliced medium thick

1 cup fresh or frozen peas
1 1/2 cups of diced-firm tofu
1/2 clove garlic, minced
1 1/2 cups zucchini, thinly sliced
1/2 cup chopped parsley
1 teaspoon dried basil
Freshly ground pepper
Salt (optional)

In a large steamer kettle with a basket, steam the vegetables until they are about half done. If using fresh peas, steam them first, then add the carrots and potato cubes after about ten minutes, and steam them all together for ten minutes more. If using frozen peas, steam the carrots and potatoes together about 7 minutes, then add the unthawed, frozen peas and steam 3-4 minutes more. If you have any turnips, they are good in here, too. Combine the vegetables together with the cubed tofu and pour into an oiled casserole. Top with the herbs and bake, uncovered in 350° F oven for 25-30 minutes, or until vegetables are tender. Makes 2 to 4 servings.

## SAUCES AND GRAVIES

### TOMATO SAUCE

3 tablespoons olive oil
1 Tablespoon finely minced garlic
2 cups crushed tomatoes
1 teaspoon crumbled oregano
1/2 teaspoon dried rosemary
Freshly ground pepper to taste
Salt to taste, if desired
2 tablespoons finely chopped fresh basil

Heat the oil in a saucepan and add the garlic. Cook briefly, stirring. Add the tomatoes, oregano, rosemary, salt, and pepper. Bring to the boil and cook, stirring occasionally, about 15 minutes. Stir in the basil and serve hot. Makes about 1 1/2 cups.

## BASIC MEXICAN SAUCE

I make this with fresh tomatoes from my garden and then freeze it, but you can use canned tomatoes if you like. This seasoning makes a medium-hot sauce, depending upon the hotness of the peppers. If you prefer a milder sauce, omit the hot peppers. This sauce is a good, all-purpose, Mexican-style sauce that I use for enchiladas, tacos, chili, and Spanish rice. It is real time saver.

Olive Oil (about 3 tablespoons)

3 medium-sized onions, chopped

2 green peppers, chopped

1 small hot pepper, chopped or 1 small can green chilis, chopped

1 large clove garlic, minced

8 cups chopped, fresh tomatoes or 4 large cans tomatoes

Freshly ground white pepper

Salt (optional)

2 tablespoons chili powder

1 tablespoons oregano

2 teaspoon basil

Dash cumin, about 1/4 teaspoon

Dash coriander, about 1/4 teaspoon

In a very large saucepan, heat some oil (about 3 tablespoons) and saute the onions, both kinds of peppers, and the garlic until the onion is soft and clear. You can brown the onion slightly. Add the fresh or canned tomatoes and the seasonings, and cook for about 2 hours, stirring frequently. You do not want the sauce to be thick like spaghetti sauce, and the tomatoes should remain in little chunks. If using fresh hot peppers, taste them first to see how hot they are. This recipe makes about three quarts after it is cooled down.

## HOMEMADE KETCHUP (CATSUP)

1 6 oz. can tomato paste

1/2 teaspoon onion powder

1/4 teaspoon garlic powder, optional or add herbs or spices of your choice

1/2 teaspoon cayenne

Mix well. Thin with water, if desired.

## CASHEW GRAVY

1 cup water
1/4 cup cashew nuts or pieces
1 tablespoon arrowroot starch or 2 tablespoons flour
1 teaspoon each of kelp, onion powder, and Vegebase
1 teaspoon safflower oil
1/4 to 1/2 teaspoon herbs of your choice — cardamom, celery seed powder, rosemary

Blenderize all ingredients well, about 2 minutes. Pour into saucepan and stir over heat until thickened.

## BASIC MUSHROOM SAUCE

1/2 cup canola oil
2 cups sliced fresh mushrooms
1 cup whole wheat pastry flour
Freshly ground white pepper
4 cups 2% milk
2 tablespoons soy sauce

In a large saucepan, melt half the butter (1/4 cup). Add the fresh mushrooms and cook them until they are slightly darkened, but still firm, about 3-4 minutes. Add the rest of the butter and melt it in. Add the four and the pepper and stir all together. Cook the flour until it is bubbly and smells nutty. Mix the soy sauce and milk together. Add slowly to the mushroom-flour mixture, stirring constantly. Cook over medium heat, stirring all the time, until the mixture is thickened and comes to the boil. Remove immediately. Cool and refrigerate. This sauce keeps for at least four days in the refrigerator, but I have frozen it without any reheating problems. If a frozen sauce separates, simply heat it in a double boiler, stirring while it heats, and it should incorporate.

## CHINESE SWEET MUSTARD SAUCE

2 tablespoons light soy sauce
1 teaspoon honey
1/4 teaspoon dry mustard
1/4 teaspoon onion powder

In a small bowl, combine all ingredients and blend well.

## SOY-TOMATO SAUCE

1/2 cup crushed tomatoes
1 tablespoons light soy sauce
1/2 teaspoon powdered ginger
1/4 teaspoon garlic powder

Combine all ingredients and blend well.

## SWEET AND SOUR SAUCE

3 tablespoons honey
3 tablespoons lemon juice
2 tablespoons ketchup
2 tablespoons soy sauce
1 tablespoons rice wine or sherry
1 teaspoon cornstarch (or arrowroot starch)
1 1/2 tablespoons canola oil
2 cloves garlic, minced
1 tablespoons minced ginger
4 scallions, white part minced, green part thinly sliced
4 cups thinly sliced vegetables and/or tofu

Combine the honey, lemon juice, ketchup, soy sauce, rice wine, and starch in a small bowl and stir until smooth. Heat a wok over a high flame. Swirl in the oil. Add the minced garlic, ginger, and scallion whites and stir-fry for 15 seconds, or until fragrant but not brown. Add the sliced vegetables and/or tofu and stir-fry for 1-2 minutes or until the vegetables are crispy tender. Restir the sauce in the bowl and then stir it into the wok. Bring the sauce to a boil. Stir in most of the scallion greens, reserving a few for garnish.

## CHINESE HOT SAUCE

This is a sauce for people who like their food hot. The hot bean paste is a fiery condiment made with chilis, soy beans, and spices.

> 2 tablespoons soy sauce
> 2 tablespoons rice vinegar or white vinegar
> 2 tablespoons rice wine or sherry
> 1-3 teaspoons hot bean paste (found in Chinese markets and gourmet shops)
> 1 1/2 teaspoon honey
> 1 teaspoon cornstarch or arrowroot starch
> 2 tablespoons canola oil
> 1-2 dried hot red chilies (optional)
> 6 cloves garlic, minced (2 tablespoons)
> 1 tablespoon minced ginger
> 4 scallions, white part minced, green part thinly sliced
> 4 cups thinly sliced vegetables and/or tofu

Combine the soy sauce, vinegar, rice wine or sherry, hot bean paste (or substitute), sugar or honey, and cornstarch in a small bowl and stir until the honey dissolves. Heat a wok over a high flame. Swirl in the oil. Add the dried chilies (if using) and fry until brown. Remove the chilies with a slotted spoon and discard. Add the minced garlic, ginger, and scallion whites and stir-fry for 15 seconds, or until fragrant but not brown. Add the vegetables and/or tofu and stir-fry for 1-2 minutes or until the vegetables are crispy-tender. Restir the sauce in the bowl and stir it into the wok. Bring the sauce to boil. Stir in most of the scallion greens, reserving a few for garnish.

## BLACK BEAN SAUCE

> 1/4 cup vegetable stock
> 2 tablespoons soy sauce
> 1 tablespoon rice wine or sherry

2 teaspoons honey

1/2 teaspoon sesame oil

1 teaspoon cornstarch (or arrowroot)

1 1/2 tablespoons canola oil

1 tablespoon minced garlic

1 tablespoon minced ginger

1 to 2 fresh hot chilies, seeded and minced (for a hotter stir-fry, leave the seeds in)

4 scallions, white part minced, green part thinly sliced

2 tablespoons cooked black beans

4 cups thinly sliced vegetables and/or tofu

Combine the vegetable stock, soy sauce, rice wine sherry, or sesame oil, and cornstarch (or arrowroot) in a small bowl and stir until the honey dissolves. Heat a wok over a high flame. Swirl in the oil. Add the minced garlic, ginger, chilies, and scallion whites and the black beans and stir-fry for 15 seconds, or until fragrant but not brown. Add the vegetables and/or tofu and stir-fry for 1-2 minutes, or until the vegetables are crispy-tender. Restir the sauce in the bowl and stir it into the stirfry. Bring the sauce to a boil and stir it into the stir- fry. Bring the sauce to a boil. Stir in most of the scallion greens, reserving a few for garnish.

# DESSERTS

## PEAR AND APPLE COMPOTE

Makes about 10 cups.

1/4 cup fresh lemon juice (2 lemons)

6 large ripe but firm Anjou or Bartlett pears (about 3 pounds)

4 Granny Smith or other tart cooking apples (about 2 pounds)

1/2 cup maple syrup (or less if you like it less sweet)

1 cinnamon stick

1 small vanilla bean, split in half lengthwise

1 tablespoon of any fruit juice sweetened fruit spread

2 teaspoons finely grated lemon organically grown lemon peel

1. Fill a stainless steal or Pyrex pot with enough boiling water to cover 1 inch of the bottom of the pot.
2. Add pears and apples to the boiling water and cover. Cover this mixture for no more than two or three minutes.
3. Add the rest of the ingredients.
4. Cook for another five minutes.
5. Serve hot or chilled.

## TOFU PROTEIN POPS

1 pound medium tofu
1/2 cup frozen juice concentrate
1/4 cup honey
1 1/2 teaspoon vanilla

Blend all ingredients until smooth. Pour into standard popsicle molds. Freeze solid. Each popsicle contains 2 1/2 grams protein. Makes 8 pops.

## TOFU RASPBERRY PUDDING

1/2 pound medium tofu
1/2 teaspoon alcohol-free vanilla extract
2 tablespoons lemon juice
1 10 oz. package frozen raspberries
1 ripe banana mashed
1/2 cup honey

Thaw and drain raspberries. Blend all ingredients until creamy. Chill and serve. Makes 3 servings.

# SALAD DRESSINGS

## CREAMY TOFU DIPS & DRESSINGS

1/2 pound tofu, cut up
1 1/2 tablespoons cider vinegar
3 tablespoons olive or safflower oil

1/4 to 1/2 teaspoon salt or 1/2 teaspoon soy sauce

Blend all ingredients in blender until smooth, keep refrigerated.

## TOFU GARLIC DRESSING

1/2 pound medium tofu
1 cup buttermilk
1 small clove garlic pressed
1/2 cup eggless, low-fat tofu-based mayonnaise (available at your health food store)
3/4 teaspoon Vegebase
1/2 teaspoon parsley
a pinch of cayenne pepper
1 tablespoons lemon juice

Blend all ingredients in blender until smooth. Keep refrigerated. Makes 1 1/2 cups.

## TOFU-BLUE CHEESE DRESSING

4 oz. medium tofu
3 oz. blue cheese or Roquefort
1/2 cup eggless, low-fat tofu-based mayonnaise (available at your health food store)
1/2 cup finely minced onion
1/2 cup distilled water
Low sodium soy sauce to taste.

Add remaining ingredients. Mix well, refrigerate. Makes 1 cup.

## SPA DRESSINGS

These dressings are often served at The New Age Health Spa in New York where I occasionally lecture. With all spa dressings; blend all ingredients in blender until smooth. Keep refrigerated.

## RED GARLIC

2 fresh tomatoes
1/4 cup chopped onion
1 tablespoon clove garlic
1/4 cup red wine vinegar
1/2 cup chopped basil
chopped parsley

## TART TAHINI

2 cups water
2 cups tahini
1/4 cup lemon juice
2 cloves garlic
1/4 cup tamari

## CREAMY MUSTARD

1 medium cucumber, peeled
1 cup low-fat yogurt
1 scallion
Juice of 1/2 lemon
1/4 cup olive oil
1 tablespoon Dijon mustard
Fresh parsley and dill
2 cloves garlic*

*Substitute basil or scallion for creamy basil or creamy scallion

## GREEN GARLIC

2 cucumber
1 cup soy mayonnaise
1/2 onion

2 cloves garlic
3 scallions
1/2 bunch dill
1/2 bunch parsley
1 tablespoon dijon mustard
1 tablespoon soy sauce
1 cup lemon juice

## SWEET DILL

2 tablespoons dijon mustard
1/4 cup apple cider vinegar
1 clove garlic
1/4 cup honey
1/2 cup water
fresh parsley and dill
dash cayenne pepper

## GINGER PEANUT

1 cup canola oil
1 cup water
2 tablespoons fresh
lemon juice
2 tablespoons honey
2 tablespoons grated ginger
1 clove garlic
1/4 cup natural
peanut butter
chopped parsley

With all spa dressings; blend all ingredients in blender until smooth.
Keep refrigerated.

## TABLE I
### Essential Amino Acid Content of Foods (as milligrams per 100 grams 3½ oz. of edible portion)

| Food | Tryptophan | Threonine | Isoleucine | Leucine | Lysine | Methionine | Phenylalanine | Valine | Histidine |
|---|---|---|---|---|---|---|---|---|---|
| **GRAINS** | | | | | | | | | |
| Barley | 160 | 433 | 545 | 889 | 433 | 184 | 661 | 643 | 239 |
| Buckwheat flour, dark | 165 | 461 | 440 | 683 | 687 | 206 | 442 | 607 | 256 |
| Buckwheat flour, light | 90 | 252 | 241 | 374 | 376 | 113 | 242 | 332 | 140 |
| Corn | | | | | | | | | |
|   Field, whole | 61 | 398 | 462 | 1296 | 288 | 186 | 454 | 510 | 206 |
|   Cornmeal, whole grain | 56 | 367 | 425 | 1192 | 265 | 171 | 418 | 470 | 190 |
|   Cornmeal, degermed | 48 | 315 | 365 | 1024 | 228 | 147 | 359 | 403 | 163 |
|   Hominy | 84 | 316 | 349 | 810 | 358 | 99 | 333 | 398 | 203 |
| Millet, pearl | 248 | 456 | 635 | 1746 | 383 | 270 | 506 | 682 | 240 |
| Millet, foxtail | 103 | 323 | 790 | 1737 | 218 | 291 | 697 | 717 | 218 |
| Oatmeal and rolled oats | 183 | 470 | 733 | 1065 | 521 | 209 | 758 | 845 | 261 |
| Rice, brown | 81 | 294 | 352 | 646 | 296 | 135 | 377 | 524 | 126 |
| Rice, white and converted | 82 | 298 | 356 | 655 | 300 | 137 | 382 | 531 | 128 |
| Rye, whole grain | 137 | 448 | 515 | 813 | 494 | 191 | 571 | 631 | 276 |
| Rye flour, medium | 129 | 422 | 485 | 766 | 465 | 180 | 538 | 594 | 260 |
| Rye flour, light | 106 | 348 | 400 | 632 | 384 | 148 | 443 | 490 | 214 |
| Sorghum | 123 | 394 | 598 | 1767 | 299 | 190 | 547 | 628 | 211 |
| Wheat whole grain, hard red spring | 173 | 403 | 607 | 939 | 384 | 214 | 691 | 648 | 286 |
| Wheat flour, whole grain | 164 | 383 | 577 | 892 | 365 | 203 | 657 | 616 | 271 |
| Wheat flour, white all-purpose | 129 | 302 | 483 | 809 | 239 | 138 | 577 | 453 | 210 |
| Wheat germ | 265 | 1343 | 1177 | 1708 | 1534 | 404 | 908 | 1364 | 687 |

278

Source: Figures are from *Amino Acid Content of Foods*, Home Economics Research Report No. 4 (Washington, D.C.: U.S. Department of Agriculture, 1968).

## LEGUMES

| | | | | | | | | | |
|---|---|---|---|---|---|---|---|---|---|
| Pinto beans | 213 | 997 | 1306 | 1976 | 1708 | 232 | 1270 | 1395 | 655 |
| Kidney beans | 214 | 1002 | 1312 | 1985 | 1715 | 233 | 1275 | 1401 | 658 |
| Navy beans | 199 | 928 | 1216 | 1839 | 1589 | 216 | 1181 | 1298 | 609 |
| Chickpeas (garbanzos) | 170 | 739 | 1195 | 1538 | 1434 | 276 | 1012 | 1025 | 559 |
| Cowpeas (black-eyed peas) | 220 | 901 | 1110 | 1715 | 1491 | 352 | 1198 | 1293 | 692 |
| Lentils | 216 | 896 | 1316 | 1760 | 1528 | 180 | 1104 | 1360 | 548 |
| Lima beans | 195 | 980 | 1199 | 1722 | 1378 | 331 | 1222 | 1298 | 669 |
| Peanuts | 340 | 828 | 1266 | 1872 | 1099 | 271 | 1557 | 1532 | 749 |
| Peanut flour | 647 | 1575 | 2410 | 3563 | 2091 | 516 | 2963 | 2916 | 1425 |
| Dried whole peas | 251 | 918 | 1340 | 1969 | 1744 | 286 | 1200 | 1333 | 651 |
| Split peas | 259 | 945 | 1380 | 2027 | 1795 | 294 | 1235 | 1372 | 670 |
| Soybeans | 526 | 1504 | 2054 | 2946 | 2414 | 513 | 1889 | 2005 | 911 |
| Soy flour, grits, full fat | 541 | 1547 | 2112 | 3030 | 2483 | 528 | 1943 | 2062 | 937 |
| Soybean sprouts | — | 159 | 225 | 265 | 211 | 45 | 186 | 225 | 133 |

## NUTS AND SEEDS

| | | | | | | | | | |
|---|---|---|---|---|---|---|---|---|---|
| Almonds | 176 | 610 | 873 | 1454 | 582 | 259 | 1146 | 1124 | 517 |
| Brazil nuts | 187 | 422 | 593 | 1129 | 443 | 941 | 617 | 823 | 367 |
| Cashews | 471 | 737 | 1222 | 1522 | 792 | 353 | 946 | 1592 | 415 |
| Coconut | 33 | 129 | 180 | 269 | 152 | 71 | 174 | 212 | 69 |
| Coconut meal | 199 | 770 | 1076 | 1605 | 908 | 421 | 1038 | 1268 | 414 |
| Filberts | 211 | 415 | 853 | 939 | 417 | 139 | 537 | 934 | 288 |
| Pecans | 138 | 389 | 553 | 773 | 435 | 153 | 564 | 525 | 273 |
| Pumpkin seeds | 560 | 933 | 1737 | 2437 | 1411 | 577 | 1749 | 1679 | 711 |
| Safflower seed meal | 675 | 1462 | 1914 | 2740 | 1525 | 731 | 2605 | 2446 | 985 |
| Sesame seed | 331 | 707 | 951 | 1679 | 583 | 637 | 1457 | 885 | 441 |
| Sesame seed meal | 573 | 1223 | 1645 | 2905 | 1008 | 1103 | 2521 | 1531 | 763 |
| Sunflower seed | 343 | 911 | 1276 | 1736 | 868 | 443 | 1220 | 1354 | 586 |
| Sunflower seed meal | 589 | 1565 | 2191 | 2981 | 1491 | 760 | 2094 | 2325 | 1006 |
| Walnuts | 175 | 589 | 767 | 1228 | 441 | 306 | 767 | 974 | 405 |

## TABLE II
### Composition of Foods (100 grams, edible portion)

| Food | Water | Food Energy | Protein | Fat | Carbohydrate Total | Fiber | Ash | Calcium | Phosphorus | Iron | Sodium | Potassium | Vitamin A | Thiamine | Riboflavin | Niacin | Ascorbic Acid |
|---|---|---|---|---|---|---|---|---|---|---|---|---|---|---|---|---|---|
| | Percent | Calories | | | Grams | | | | | Milligrams | | | IU | | Milligrams | | |
| **GRAINS AND GRAIN PRODUCTS** | | | | | | | | | | | | | | | | | |
| Barley, | | | | | | | | | | | | | | | | | |
| Pearled, light | 11.1 | 349 | 8.2 | 1.0 | 78.8 | .5 | .9 | 16 | 189 | 2.0 | 3 | 160 | (0) | .12 | .05 | 3.1 | (0) |
| Pearled, Scotch | 10.8 | 348 | 9.6 | 1.1 | 77.2 | .9 | 1.3 | 34 | 290 | 2.7 | — | 296 | (0) | .21 | .07 | 3.7 | (0) |
| Buckwheat | | | | | | | | | | | | | | | | | |
| Whole grain | 11.0 | 335 | 11.7 | 2.4 | 72.9 | 9.9 | 2.0 | 114 | 282 | 3.1 | — | 448 | (0) | .60 | — | 4.4 | (0) |
| Flour, dark | 12.0 | 333 | 11.7 | 2.5 | 72.0 | 1.6 | 1.8 | 33 | 347 | 2.8 | — | — | (0) | .58 | .15 | 2.9 | (0) |
| Flour, light | 12.0 | 347 | 6.4 | 1.2 | 79.5 | .5 | .9 | 11 | 88 | 1.0 | — | 320 | (0) | .08 | (.04) | (.4) | (0) |
| Corn | | | | | | | | | | | | | | | | | |
| Field, raw dried | 13.8 | 348 | 8.9 | 3.9 | 72.2 | 2.0 | 1.2 | 22 | 268 | 2.1 | 1 | 284 | 490* | .37 | .12 | 2.2 | (0) |
| Sweet, yellow raw | 72.7 | 96 | 3.5 | 1.0 | 22.1 | .7 | .7 | 3 | 111 | .7 | trace | 280 | 400* | .15 | .12 | 1.7 | 12 |
| Cooked, boiled, drained (cut before cooking) | 76.5 | 83 | 3.2 | 1.0 | 18.8 | .7 | .5 | 3 | 89 | .6 | trace | 165 | 400* | .11 | .10 | 1.3 | 7 |
| Cooked on cob | 74.1 | 91 | 3.3 | 1.0 | 21.0 | .7 | .6 | 3 | 89 | .6 | trace | 196 | 400* | .12 | .10 | 1.4 | 9 |
| Corn flour | 12.0 | 368 | 7.8 | 2.6 | 76.8 | .7 | .8 | 6 | (164) | 1.8 | (1) | — | 340* | .20 | .06 | 1.4 | (0) |
| Degermed corn grits, enriched, raw | 12.0 | 362 | 8.7 | .8 | 78.1 | .4 | .4 | .4 | 73 | 2.9 | 1 | 80 | 440* | .44 | .26 | 3.5 | (0) |

Figures are from *Agriculture Handbook No. 8, Composition of Foods* (Washington, D.C.: Agricultural Research Service, United States Dept. of Agriculture, unless otherwise noted).

Note: Numbers in parentheses denote values inputed—usually from another form of the same or similar food. Zero in parentheses indicates that the amount of a constituent probably is none or is too small to measure. Dashes denote lack of reliable data for a constituent believed to be present in measurable amount.

*Based on yellow varieties of corn.

**Nitrogen-free extract.

[1]From J.H. Hulse, and E.M. Laing, *Nutritive Value Of Triticale Protein*. (Ottawa: International Development Research Center, 1974).

[2]From K. Lorenz, The History, Development, and Utilization of Triticale. *CRC Critical Reviews in Food Technology*, 1974.

| Food | Water (%) | Food energy (cal.) | Protein (g) | Fat (g) | Carbohydrate (g) | Fiber (g) | Ash (g) | Calcium (mg) | Phosphorus (mg) | Iron (mg) | Sodium (mg) | Potassium (mg) | Vitamin A (I.U.) | Thiamine (mg) | Riboflavin (mg) | Niacin (mg) | Ascorbic acid (mg) |
|---|---|---|---|---|---|---|---|---|---|---|---|---|---|---|---|---|---|
| Degermed corn grits, unenriched, raw | 12.0 | 362 | 8.7 | .8 | 78.1 | .4 | .4 | 4 | 73 | .0 | - | 80 | 440* | .13 | .04 | 1.2 | (0) |
| Cornmeal, whole grain, (unbolted) | 12.0 | 355 | 9.2 | 3.9 | 73.7 | 1.6 | 1.2 | 20 | 256 | 2.4 | (1) | (284) | 510* | .38 | .11 | 2.0 | (0) |
| Cornmeal, bolted | 12.0 | 362 | 9.0 | 3.4 | 74.5 | 1.0 | 1.1 | (17) | (223) | 1.8 | (1) | (248) | 480* | .30 | .08 | 1.9 | (0) |
| Cornmeal, degermed, enriched | 12.0 | 364 | 7.9 | 1.2 | 78.4 | .6 | .5 | 6 | 99 | 2.9 | 1 | 120 | 440* | .44 | .26 | 3.5 | (0) |
| Cornmeal, degermed, unenriched | 12.0 | 364 | 7.9 | 1.2 | 78.4 | .6 | .5 | 6 | 99 | 1.1 | 1 | 120 | 440* | .14 | .05 | 1.0 | (0) |
| Millet (proso, broomcorn, hog millet), whole grain | 11.8 | 327 | 9.9 | 2.9 | 72.9 | 3.2 | 2.5 | 20 | 311 | 6.8 | — | 430 | (0) | .73 | .38 | 2.3 | (0) |
| Rolled oats, dry | 8.3 | 390 | 14.2 | 7.4 | 68.2 | 1.2 | 1.9 | 53 | 405 | 4.5 | 2 | 352 | (0) | .60 | .14 | 1.0 | (0) |
| Rolled oats, cooked | 86.5 | 55 | 2.0 | 1.0 | 9.7 | .2 | .8 | 9 | 57 | .6 | 218 | 61 | (0) | .08 | .02 | .1 | (0) |
| Rice, Brown, raw | 12.0 | 360 | 7.5 | 1.9 | 77.4 | .9 | 1.2 | 32 | 221 | 1.6 | 9 | 214 | (0) | .34 | .05 | 4.7 | (0) |
| Brown, cooked | 70.3 | 119 | 2.5 | .6 | 25.5 | .3 | 1.1 | 12 | 73 | .5 | 282 | 70 | (0) | .09 | .02 | 1.4 | (0) |
| White enriched, raw | 12.0 | 363 | 6.7 | .4 | 80.4 | .3 | .5 | 24 | 94 | 2.9 | 5 | 92 | (0) | .44 | .26 | 3.5 | (0) |
| White enriched, cooked | 72.6 | 109 | 2.0 | .1 | 24.2 | .1 | 1.1 | 10 | 28 | .9 | 374 | 28 | (0) | .11 | .01 | 1.0 | (0) |
| White parboiled long grain, raw | 10.3 | 369 | 7.4 | .3 | 81.3 | .2 | .7 | 60 | 200 | 2.9 | 9 | 150 | (0) | .44 | .26 | 3.5 | (0) |
| White parboiled long grain, cooked | 73.4 | 106 | 2.1 | .1 | 23.3 | .1 | 1.1 | 19 | 57 | .8 | 9 | 43 | (0) | .11 | .07 | 1.2 | (0) |
| Rice, precooked (instant), dry | 9.6 | 374 | 7.5 | .2 | 82.5 | .4 | .2 | 5 | 65 | 2.9 | 358 | — | (0) | .44 | .26 | 3.5 | (0) |
| Rice, precooked ready-to-serve | 72.9 | 109 | 2.2 | trace | 24.2 | .1 | .7 | 3 | 19 | .8 | 273 | trace | (0) | .13 | .07 | 1.0 | (0) |
| Rye, Whole grain | 11.0 | 334 | 12.1 | 1.7 | 73.4 | 2.0 | 1.8 | (38) | 376 | 3.7 | (1) | 467 | (0) | .43 | .22 | 1.6 | (0) |
| Light flour | 11.0 | 357 | 9.4 | 1.0 | 77.9 | .4 | .7 | 22 | 185 | 1.1 | (1) | 156 | (0) | .15 | .07 | .6 | (0) |
| Med. flour | 11.0 | 350 | 11.4 | 1.7 | 74.8 | 1.0 | 1.1 | (27) | 262 | 2.6 | (1) | 203 | (0) | .30 | .12 | 2.5 | (0) |
| Dark flour | 11.0 | 327 | 16.3 | 2.6 | 68.1 | 2.4 | 2.0 | 54 | (536) | 4.5 | 1 | 860 | (0) | .61 | .22 | 2.7 | (0) |
| Sorghum grain | 11.0 | 332 | 11.0 | 3.3 | 73.0 | 1.7 | 1.7 | 28 | 287 | 4.4 | — | 350 | (0) | .38 | .15 | 3.9 | (0) |

## TABLE II
### Composition of Foods (100 grams, edible portion)

| Food | Water | Food Energy | Protein | Fat | Carbohydrate Total | Fiber | Ash | Calcium | Phosphorus | Iron | Sodium | Potassium | Vitamin A | Thiamine | Riboflavin | Niacin | Ascorbic Acid |
|---|---|---|---|---|---|---|---|---|---|---|---|---|---|---|---|---|---|
| | Per-cent | Cal-ories | Grams | Grams | Grams | Grams | Grams | Milligrams | Milligrams | Milligrams | Milligrams | Milligrams | IU | Milligrams | Milligrams | Milligrams | Milligrams |
| **GRAINS AND GRAIN PRODUCTS (cont.)** | | | | | | | | | | | | | | | | | |
| Triticale[1,2] | 8–16 | 360 | 10.8–18.6 | 3.2–4.6 | 71.4–81.0** | 3.1 | 1.9–2.3 | 27–36 | 437–534 | 4.5–5.7 | 2.9–5.7 | 358–508 | — | — | — | — | — |
| Wheat, whole grain | | | | | | | | | | | | | | | | | |
| Hard red spring | 13.0 | 330 | 14.0 | 2.2 | 69.1 | 2.3 | 1.7 | 36 | 383 | 3.1 | (3) | 370 | (0) | .57 | .12 | 4.3 | (0) |
| Hard red winter | 12.5 | 330 | 12.3 | 1.8 | 71.7 | 2.3 | 1.7 | 46 | 354 | 3.4 | (3) | 370 | (0) | .52 | .12 | 4.3 | (0) |
| Soft red winter | 14.0 | 326 | 10.2 | 2.0 | 72.1 | 2.3 | 1.7 | 42 | 400 | 3.5 | (3) | 376 | (0) | .43 | .11 | (3.6) | (0) |
| White | 11.5 | 335 | 9.4 | 2.0 | 75.4 | 1.9 | 1.7 | 36 | 394 | 3.0 | (3) | 390 | (0) | .53 | .12 | 5.3 | (0) |
| Durum | 13.0 | 332 | 12.7 | 2.5 | 70.1 | 1.8 | 1.7 | 37 | 386 | 4.3 | (3) | 435 | (0) | .66 | .12 | (4.4) | (0) |
| Whole wheat flour (hard wheat) | 12.0 | 333 | 13.3 | 2.0 | 71.0 | 2.3 | 1.7 | 41 | 372 | 3.3 | 3 | 370 | (0) | .55 | .12 | 4.3 | (0) |
| Enriched white flour (all purpose) | 12.0 | 364 | 10.5 | 1.0 | 76.1 | .3 | .43 | 16 | 87 | 2.9 | 2 | 95 | (0) | .44 | .26 | 3.5 | (0) |
| Bulgur Club wheat, dry | 9.0 | 359 | 8.7 | 1.4 | 79.5 | 1.7 | 1.4 | 30 | 319 | 4.7 | — | 262 | (0) | .30 | .10 | (4.2) | (0) |
| Hard red winter wheat, dry | 10.0 | 354 | 11.2 | 1.5 | 75.7 | 1.7 | 1.6 | 29 | 338 | 3.7 | — | 229 | (0) | .28 | .14 | 4.5 | (0) |
| White wheat, dry | (9.0) | 357 | 10.3 | 1.2 | 78.1 | 1.3 | 1.4 | 36 | 300 | (4.7) | — | 310 | (0) | (.30) | (.10) | (4.2) | (0) |
| Canned, unseasoned | 56.0 | 168 | 6.2 | .7 | 35.0 | .8 | 2.1 | 20 | 200 | 1.3 | 599 | 87 | (0) | .05 | .03 | 2.4 | (0) |
| Canned, seasoned | 56.0 | 182 | 6.2 | 3.3 | 32.8 | .8 | 1.7 | 20 | 195 | 1.4 | 460 | 112 | (0) | .06 | .04 | 3.0 | (0) |
| Wild rice, raw | 8.5 | 353 | 14.1 | .7 | 75.3 | 1.0 | 1.4 | 19 | 339 | 4.2 | 7 | 220 | (0) | .45 | .63 | 6.2 | (0) |
| **NUTS AND SEEDS** | | | | | | | | | | | | | | | | | |
| Almonds | 4.7 | 598 | 18.6 | 54.2 | 19.5 | 2.6 | 3.0 | 234 | 504 | 4.7 | 4 | 773 | 0 | .24 | .92 | 3.5 | tr |
| Beechnuts | 6.6 | 568 | 19.4 | 50.0 | 20.3 | 3.7 | 3.7 | — | — | — | — | — | — | — | — | — | — |
| Brazilnuts | 4.6 | 654 | 14.3 | 66.9 | 10.9 | 3.1 | 3.3 | 186 | 693 | 3.4 | 1 | 715 | tr | .96 | .12 | 1.6 | — |
| Butternuts | 3.8 | 629 | 23.7 | 61.2 | 8.4 | — | 2.9 | — | — | 6.8 | — | — | — | — | — | — | — |
| Cashews | 5.2 | 561 | 17.2 | 45.7 | 29.3 | 1.4 | 2.6 | 38 | 373 | 3.8 | 15 | 464 | 100 | .43 | .25 | 1.8 | — |

282

| Food | | | | | | | | | | | | | | | | |
|---|---|---|---|---|---|---|---|---|---|---|---|---|---|---|---|---|
| Chestnuts, fresh | 52.5 | 194 | 2.9 | 1.5 | 42.1 | 1.1 | 1.0 | 27 | 88 | 1.7 | 6 | 454 | — | .22 | .22 | .6 | — |
| Chestnuts, dried | 8.4 | 377 | 6.7 | 4.1 | 78.6 | 2.5 | 2.2 | 52 | 162 | 3.3 | 12 | 875 | — | .32 | .38 | 1.2 | — |
| Hickory nuts | 3.3 | 673 | 13.2 | 68.7 | 12.8 | 1.9 | 2.0 | tr | 360 | 2.4 | — | — | 0 | — | — | — | 0 |
| Macadamia nuts | 3.0 | 691 | 7.8 | 71.6 | 15.9 | 2.5 | 1.7 | 48 | 161 | 2.0 | tr | 264 | 130 | .34 | .11 | 1.3 | 2 |
| Pecans | 3.4 | 687 | 9.2 | 71.2 | 14.6 | 2.3 | 1.6 | 73 | 289 | 2.4 | — | 603 | — | .86 | .13 | .9 | tr |
| Pignolias | 5.6 | 552 | 31.1 | 47.4 | 11.6 | .9 | 4.3 | — | — | — | — | — | 30 | .62 | .23 | 4.5 | 0 |
| Piñon | 3.1 | 635 | 13.0 | 60.5 | 20.5 | 1.1 | 2.9 | 12 | 604 | 5.2 | — | 972 | 230 | 1.28 | .19 | 1.4 | — |
| Pistachios | 5.3 | 594 | 19.3 | 53.7 | 19.0 | 1.9 | 2.7 | 131 | 500 | 7.3 | — | — | 70 | .67 | — | 2.4 | — |
| Pumpkin and squash seed kernels, dry | 4.4 | 553 | 29.0 | 46.7 | 15.0 | 1.9 | 4.9 | 51 | 1,144 | 11.2 | — | — | — | .24 | — | — | 0 |
| Safflower seed kernels, dry | 5.0 | 615 | 19.1 | 59.5 | 12.4 | — | 4.0 | — | — | — | 60 | 725 | 30 | — | .24 | — | 0 |
| Sesame seeds dry, whole | 5.4 | 563 | 18.6 | 49.1 | 21.6 | 6.3 | 5.3 | 1,160 | 616 | 10.5 | — | — | — | .98 | .13 | 5.4 | — |
| Seseme seeds hulled | 5.5 | 582 | 18.2 | 53.4 | 17.6 | 2.4 | 5.3 | 110 | 592 | 2.4 | 30 | 920 | 50 | .18 | .23 | 5.4 | — |
| Sunflower seed kernels, dry | 4.8 | 560 | 24.0 | 47.3 | 19.9 | 3.8 | 4.0 | 120 | 837 | 7.1 | — | 920 | 300 | 1.96 | .11 | 5.4 | 2 |
| Black walnuts | 3.1 | 628 | 20.5 | 59.3 | 14.8 | 1.7 | 2.3 | tr | 570 | 6.0 | 3 | 460 | 30 | .22 | .13 | .7 | — |
| English or Persian walnuts | 3.5 | 651 | 14.8 | 64.0 | 15.8 | 2.1 | 1.9 | 99 | 380 | 3.1 | 2 | 450 | 0 | .33 | .22 | .9 | 0 |
| **LEGUMES** | | | | | | | | | | | | | | | | | |
| Beans, dry | | | | | | | | | | | | | | | | | |
| White, raw | 10.9 | 340 | 22.3 | 1.6 | 61.3 | 4.3 | 3.9 | 144 | 425 | 7.8 | 19 | 1,196 | 0 | .65 | .07 | 2.4 | — |
| White, cooked | 69.0 | 118 | 7.8 | .6 | 21.2 | 1.5 | 1.4 | 50 | 148 | 2.7 | 7 | 416 | 0 | .14 | .20 | .7 | — |
| Red, raw | 10.4 | 343 | 22.5 | 1.5 | 61.9 | 4.2 | 3.7 | 110 | 406 | 6.9 | 10 | 984 | 20 | .51 | .06 | 2.3 | — |
| Red, cooked | 69.0 | 118 | 7.8 | .5 | 21.4 | 1.5 | 1.3 | 38 | 140 | 2.4 | 3 | 340 | trace | .11 | .21 | .7 | — |
| Pinto, calico, red Mexican, raw | 8.3 | 349 | 22.9 | 1.2 | 63.7 | 4.3 | 3.9 | 135 | 457 | 6.4 | 10 | 984 | — | .84 | .20 | 2.2 | — |
| Other (incl black, brown, Bayo) raw | 11.2 | 339 | 22.3 | 1.5 | 61.2 | 4.4 | 3.8 | 135 | 420 | 7.9 | 25 | 1,038 | 30 | .55 | .17 | 2.2 | — |
| Lima, dry, raw | 10.3 | 345 | 20.4 | 1.6 | 64.0 | 4.3 | 3.7 | 72 | 385 | 7.8 | 4 | 1,529 | tr | .48 | .06 | 1.9 | — |
| Lima, cooked | 64.1 | 138 | 8.2 | .6 | 25.6 | 1.7 | 1.5 | 29 | 154 | 3.1 | 2 | 612 | — | .13 | .21 | .7 | — |
| Mung, dry, raw | 10.7 | 340 | 24.2 | 1.3 | 60.3 | 4.4 | 3.5 | 118 | 340 | 7.7 | 6 | 1,028 | 80 | .38 | .13 | 2.6 | — |
| Mung beans, sprouted, raw | 88.8 | 35 | 3.8 | .2 | 6.6 | .7 | .6 | 19 | 64 | 1.3 | 5 | 223 | 20 | .13 | .31 | .8 | 19 |
| Soybeans dry, raw | 10.0 | 403 | 34.1 | 17.7 | 33.5 | 4.9 | 4.7 | 226 | 554 | 8.4 | 5 | 1,677 | 80 | 1.10 | .09 | 2.2 | — |
| Soybeans, cooked | 71.0 | 130 | 11.0 | 5.7 | 10.8 | 1.6 | 1.5 | 73 | 179 | 2.7 | 2 | 540 | 30 | .21 | .10 | .6 | 0 |
| Soybeans, miso | 53.0 | 171 | 10.5 | 4.6 | 23.5 | 2.3 | 8.4 | 68 | 309 | 1.7 | 2,950 | 334 | 40 | .06 | .20 | .3 | 0 |
| Soybeans, sprout, raw | 86.3 | 46 | 6.2 | 1.4 | 5.3 | .8 | .8 | 48 | 67 | 1.0 | — | — | 80 | .23 | — | .8 | 13 |

283

**TABLE II** Composition of Foods *(continued)*

| Food | Water Per-cent | Food Energy Cal-ories | Protein | Fat | Carbohydrate Total | Carbohydrate Fiber | Ash | Cal-cium | Phos-phorus | Iron | Sodium | Potas-sium | Vitamin A IU | Thia-mine | Ribo-flavin | Niacin | Ascor-bic Acid |
|---|---|---|---|---|---|---|---|---|---|---|---|---|---|---|---|---|---|
| | | | Grams | | | | | Milligrams | | | | | IU | Milligrams | | | |
| **LEGUMES (cont.)** | | | | | | | | | | | | | | | | | |
| Soybeans, tofu | 84.8 | 72 | 7.8 | 4.2 | 2.4 | .1 | .8 | 128 | 126 | 1.9 | 7 | 42 | 0 | .06 | .03 | .1 | 0 |
| Soyflour, full fat | 8.0 | 421 | 36.7 | 20.3 | 30.4 | 2.4 | 4.6 | 199 | 558 | 8.4 | 1 | 1,660 | 110 | .85 | .31 | 2.1 | 0 |
| Soyflour, defatted | 8.0 | 326 | 47.0 | .9 | 38.1 | 2.3 | 6.0 | 265 | 655 | 11.1 | 1 | 1,820 | 40 | 1.09 | .34 | 2.6 | — |
| Carob flour (St. Johns bread) | 11.2 | 180 | 4.5 | 1.4 | 80.7 | 7.7 | 2.2 | 352 | 81 | — | — | — | — | — | — | — | — |
| Chick-peas (garbanzos), dry raw | 10.7 | 360 | 20.5 | 4.8 | 61.0 | 5.0 | 3.0 | 150 | 133 | 6.9 | 26 | 797 | 50 | .31 | .15 | 2.0 | — |
| Cowpeas (black-eyed peas) dry, raw | 10.5 | 343 | 22.8 | 1.5 | 61.7 | 4.4 | 3.5 | 74 | 426 | 5.8 | 35 | 1,024 | 30 | 1.05 | .21 | 2.2 | — |
| Cowpeas, dry, cooked | 80.0 | 76 | 5.1 | .3 | 13.8 | 1.0 | .8 | 17 | 95 | 1.3 | 8 | 229 | 10 | .16 | .04 | .4 | — |
| Lentils, dry, raw | 11.1 | 340 | 24.7 | 1.1 | 60.1 | 3.9 | 3.0 | 79 | 377 | 6.8 | 30 | 790 | 60 | .37 | .22 | 2.0 | — |
| Lentils, dry cooked | 72.0 | 106 | 7.8 | tr | 19.3 | 1.2 | .9 | 25 | 119 | 2.1 | — | 249 | 20 | .07 | .06 | .6 | 0 |
| Peanuts | | | | | | | | | | | | | | | | | |
| Raw, with skins | 5.6 | 564 | 26.0 | 47.5 | 18.6 | 2.4 | 2.3 | 69 | 401 | 2.1 | 5 | 674 | — | 1.14 | .13 | 17.2 | 0 |
| Raw, without skins | 5.4 | 568 | 26.3 | 48.4 | 17.6 | 1.9 | 2.3 | 59 | 409 | 2.0 | 5 | 674 | 0 | .99 | .13 | 15.8 | 0 |
| Boiled | 36.4 | 376 | 15.5 | 31.5 | 14.5 | 1.8 | 2.1 | 43 | 181 | 1.3 | 4 | 462 | — | .48 | .08 | 10.0 | 0 |
| Roasted, with skins | 1.8 | 582 | 26.2 | 48.7 | 20.6 | 2.7 | 2.7 | 72 | 407 | | 5 | 701 | — | .32 | .13 | 17.1 | 0 |
| Roasted and salted | 1.6 | 585 | 26.0 | 49.8 | 18.8 | 2.4 | 3.8 | 74 | 401 | 3.5 | 418 | 674 | — | .32 | .13 | 17.2 | 0 |
| Flour, defatted | 7.3 | 371 | 47.9 | 9.2 | 31.5 | 2.7 | 4.1 | 104 | 720 | | 9 | 1,186 | — | .75 | .22 | 27.8 | 0 |
| Dried green peas, raw, whole | 11.7 | 340 | 24.1 | 1.3 | 60.3 | 4.9 | 2.6 | 64 | 340 | 5.1 | 35 | 1,005 | 120 | .74 | .29 | 3.0 | 0 |
| Split peas, raw, no seed coat | 9.3 | 348 | 24.2 | 1.0 | 62.7 | 1.2 | 2.8 | 33 | 268 | 5.1 | 40 | 895 | 120 | .74 | .29 | 3.0 | — |
| Cooked | 70.0 | 115 | 8.0 | .3 | 20.8 | .4 | .9 | 11 | 89 | 1.7 | 13 | 296 | 40 | .15 | .09 | .9 | — |

# HERBAL HEALING

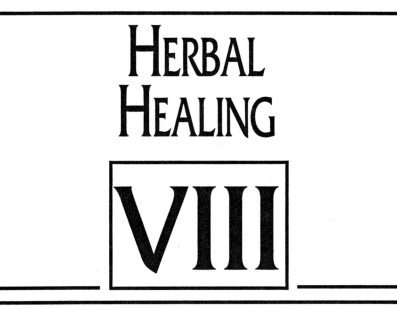

# VIII

The practice of herbal healing goes back to the dawn of man. Ancient Egyptian and Chinese texts thousands of years old have recorded the use of herbs for treating and curing various ailments of the body, mind and spirit. Many of the plants used today in herbal medicine were used and described by Dioscorides, a first century Greek physician and botanist. His reference work "De Materia Medica," was for 1,500 years the standard work on botany and therapeutic use of plants.

The use of herbal teas, extracts and powders to help rebuild sickly and weak bodies is still used by virtually every culture. Many Native American communities used herbs for medicine, dyes, poisons and food. The Aztecs used nettles regularly and early American pioneers used lovage, sage, chives, lily of the valley, peppermint, thyme, flax, pennyroyal and chamomile. The English used dandelion and the Chinese, ginseng.

Today many herbs are used in modern medicine. Though many of these herbal remedies do not have a scientific basis as to why they work, they are the basis of some well known pharmaceuticals. It was the *cinchona* tree that gave us *quinine* for the treatment of malaria, the *foxglove* plant that gave us digitalis. Other herbs that are currently used by medical doctors in one form or another include red periwinkle, mayapple, witch hazel, and ginseng.

Though there is more sophisticated research on the value of herbal medicines than ever before, most of the information about herbs used in natural healing is based on the folklore passed down from generation to generation. Over the last fifteen years the use of herbal medicines in healing has increased to an amazing level. Herbal experts cite these major reasons why herbs have gained new found popularity: (1) many people desire to return to nature; (2) they fear the side effects associated with many over-the-counter and prescription drugs; (3) they are unhappy with the high cost and impersonal style of orthodox medicine; and (4) they've discovered that Indian, African, Asian and South American cultures have used herbal medicines with great success.

## HERBS AS HEALERS

Among the most popular herbal healers used are:

*Aloe vera.* The gel of this plant may be applied topically to burns and other skin problems, and it is often taken orally as well. Aloe is often used in the southwestern United States and in Latin American for its antibacterial, antifungal and antiviral properties. In the Philippines, aloe vera gel is mixed with milk for the treatment of dysentery, intestinal infections and kidney problems. There are tribes in Zaire that use aloe for the treatment of ringworm and boils. Many healers use the aloe gel for the treatment of digestive problems, arthritis and bursitis.

*Anise (Pimpinella anisum).* Anise may be boiled in milk to relieve gas pains and colic in small children. Anise tea is very soothing to the digestive tract.

*Astragalus (Astragalus membranaceus).* This is one of the most popular tonic herbs in oriental medicine. It has been used primarily to strengthen the immune system. Any disease or disorder that involved a breakdown or weakness of the immune system would call for astragalus as part of the total healing program.

*Arnica (Arnica montana).* This herb can be used as an external tincture for sprains and bruises.

*Bayberry bark (Myrica cerifera).* An excellent gargle for sore throats, bayberry is also used to clear congestion in the nose and sinuses.

*Black cohash root (Cimicifuga racemosa).* Used to reduce menopausal symptoms. Reduces pain in childbirth. Contains estrogen like substance.

*Black walnut hulls.* Used for many skin disorders. Expels parasites.

*Blessed thistle (Juglans nigra).* Useful for relieving migraine headaches. Valuable in many gynecological disorders.

*Blue cohash (Caulophyllus thalictroides).* Regulates menstrual flow. Used for heart palpitations and hypertension.

*Burdock root (Arctium lappa).* A blood cleanser and diuretic. It is also healing to the kidneys.

*Butcher's Broom (Ruscus aculeatus).* This herb is more popular in Europe than in the United States, but it is beginning to develop a strong following among natural healers due to it's anti-clotting and anti-inflammatory properties. It is most commonly used to treat various circulatory problems.

*Capsicum (Capsicum minimum).* This is common cayenne pepper. It is a catalyst for most other herbs. It is valuable for circulation, the heart and nerves.

*Catnip (Nepeta cataris).* Useful for children with colic, soothing to the nerves. Reduces pain from spasms.

*Chamomile (Anthemis nobilis).* Sedating to the entire nervous system. Reduces teething pain in children. Chamomile is used in many formulas for reducing stress.

*Chaparral (larrea tridentata; L.divaricata).* Used in many traditional herbal cancer treatment formulas. Used for arthritis, infections, acne and other skin conditions.

*Chickweed (Stellaria madia, Cyrill).* Used for swollen testes, hemorrhoids, bronchial problems.

*Comfrey (Symphytum officinale).* Available as a root or leaves. The root is most popular. Good for diarrhea, blood in urine, coughs and colds. Used to heal ulcers.

*Damiana (Turnera diffusa, Willd.).* Sexual rejuvenator and nerve stimulant.

*Dandelion root (Taraxacum officinale, Wiggers).* When used raw, it is a powerful diuretic; good for kidney and bladder problems.

*Echinacea (Echinacea angustifolia).* Used for all fevers and infections. Excellent blood cleanser.

*Eyebright (Euphrasia officinalis).* Used internally as a tea for problems of the eye, including conjunctivitis.

*Evening Primrose (Primula vulgaris, Huds.).* The oil of this plant is very high in certain hormone-like substances known as prostaglandins. Prostaglandins have been found to bring relief to a number of medical disorders.

*Fennel (Foeniculum vulgare).* Reduces flatulence and bloating from gas. Reduces colic in children. Good for digestion.

*Fo-Ti.* Helps memory and reduces depression. (A Chinese herb).

*Garlic (Allium sativum).* Garlic is an aid in healing all systemic infections, respiratory problems and fever.

*Ginger (Zingiber officinale).* Reduces painful spasms of bowels and stomach. Used as a tea and in compresses. Ginger is one of the most popular herbs in Vietnamese medicine along with peppermint and eucalyptus.

*Ginseng (Pana quinquefolium).* Helps with nervous exhaustion, sexual function, poor circulation, loss of memory.

*Goldenseal root (Hydrastis canadensis).* One of the most popular herbs. Used to treat ulcers and most internal infections.

*Gotu kola.* Used in many nerve stimulant formulas.

*Hawthorn berries (Crataegus oxycantha).* Used for all heart problems.

*Horsetail (Equisetum arvense, Linn.).* Rich in silica. Helps skin healing and is a diuretic.

*Jojoba.* This desert shrub produces a wax-like substance (called jojoba oil) that is very similar to sperm whale oil. It is a highly versatile lubricant that is most useful in healing various skin and scalp disorders.

*Juniper berries (Juniperus communis).* Used in pancreatic, adrenal, bladder and kidney disorders. Especially useful in leucorrhea and edema.

*Licorice root (Glycyrrhiza glabra).* Soothing to the throat, licorice root contains a natural cortisone-like substance. Used for hypoglycemia, ulcers, stress and adrenal related problems.

*Lobelia (Lobelia inflata, Linn.).* The most powerful of all herbal relaxants. Reduces palpitation of the heart, fever. Note, however, this herb should be used under the direction of a skilled herbalist.

*Marsh mallow root (Althaea officinalis, Linn.).* Bathe inflamed eyes in this tea. Good for problems of the lungs, kidneys, throat and digestion, especially diarrhea.

*Myrrh (Commiphora molmol).* Usually taken as tincture. Still used by many dentists. Used for ulcers, hemorrhoids, bronchial and lung disorders.

*Parsley (Carum petroselinum).* A powerful diuretic, rich in chlorophyll. Traditionally used for all gallbladder problems and for expelling stones.

*Pau D'Arco (Taheebo).* Taheebo is the Indian name for the inner bark of the Tabebuia tree, found only in the Andes mountains. This bark has been traditionally used by the Callaway tribe (descendants of the Incas). Taheebo contains a compound called *quechua,* a powerful antibiotic with virus-killing properties. The herb can be taken as a tea or in a salve form. It has been used to reduce pain, to serve as a blood-builder, and to strengthen the immune response. Many healers claim that taheebo is effective in the treatment of candida, herpes and certain types of caner. Limited research on the herb has been conducted in the United States, though it has become a popular healing herb in the last five years.

*Peppermint(Mentha piperita).* Used for digestion and reducing fever. Use the cool tea to wash burns. It is high in tannic acid.

*Plantain (plantago major, Linn.).* Primarily used for menstrual disorders, plantain is also good for problems of the lungs, kidneys, throat and digestion especially, diarrhea.

*Psyllium (Plantago psyllium, Linn.).* Colon cleanser. Used in most detoxification programs.

*Red clover (Trifolium pratense, Linn.).* Relaxing for the nervous system. One of the best blood cleansers.

*Raspberry (Rubus idaeus, Linn.).* Relieves morning sickness in pregnancy. Strengthens the uterine wall prior to childbirth.

*Rosemary (Rosemarinus officinalis).* This pungent herb has been found in recent research to have the ability to act as an anti-oxidant and preservative in food. Because of its strong odor and taste, it cannot easily be used in all foods.

*Saffron (Crocus sativus).* Aids digestion, arthritis and muscle fatigue.

*Sage.* Gargle with this tea to relieve a sore throat and ulcers in the mouth. Reduces involuntary sexual emissions in men (spermatorrhea). Expels worms. Also used for kidney and liver problems.

*Sarsparilla (Similax officinalis).* Blood cleanser.

*Sassafrass (Sassafras variifolium).* Used to ease colic and to heal skin eruptions. It was used by Native American tribes of the northeastern United States as a spring medicine to purify the blood.

*Siberian Ginseng (Eleutherococcus Senticosus).* This is not actually ginseng, but rather it is a member of the Araliaceae family of plants. Unlike other herbs this herb is not known for any particular curative effect but instead for retroactive qualities. It is very valuable for people who are coming back from a health problem and are beginning to regain their strength.

*Skullcap (Scutellaria laterifolia, Linn.).* One of the best herbs for nervous disorders. It is used to reduce hypertension, heart problems and any problems of the central nervous system, including epilepsy.

*Slippery elm bark (Ulmus fulva).* This pleasant tasting herb was used by the native population and the early settlers in the form of poultices and liquids for the treatment of fevers and colds with cough. When treating an individual in a weak and debilitated condition, slippery elm supplies both a nutritive and gentle action on the body. Because of its mucilagenous quality, it is an ideal herb for tissue repair and is also known for its anti-inflammatory qualities.

*Thyme (Thymus vulgaris, Linn.).* Thyme can be used as an antiseptic and anti-spasmodic. Its aromatic essence is used to treat fevers and infections.

*Uva Ursi or Bearberry (Arctostaphylos uva-ursi).* Used in mature onset diabetes, kidney and bladder problems.

*Valerian root.* One of the best herbs for nervous disorders. Is used to reduce hypertension, heart problems and any problems of the central nervous system including epilepsy. Especially useful for sleep disorders.

***White oak bark.*** Used for varicose veins and hemorrhoids. Normalizes the liver, kidney and spleen.

***White willow bark (Salix alba).*** An Indian folk medicine which contains salicin, a prime ingredient in aspirin and a powerful anti-inflammatory agent, especially for arthritis.

***Yarrow.*** Used for indigestion and run down conditions. If used at the beginning of a cold, it is very soothing to the mucous membranes and may break up the illness within 24 hours.

***Yellow dock..*** Blood purifier and toner for the entire system. Very high in minerals.

***Yohimbe.*** This herb is actually the bark of a tree that grows in Africa and Mexico. It has been used historically in tribal medicine as an aphrodisiac and sexual rejuvenator as well as a general remedy for impotency and other sexual dysfunctions. This herb should be used with caution and under the guidance of a trained herbalist or physician. Yohimbe is so strong a sexual stimulant that the hydrochloride derivative is a prescription drug.

***Yucca.*** A desert plant that has shown some positive results in treating rheumatoid arthritis.

# BIBLIOGRAPHY AND REFERENTIAL READING

- Fasting For The Renewal Of Life, By Herbert M. Shelton, (Natural Hygiene Press), 1974
- Fasting: The Ultimate Diet, By Allan Cott, M.D., Published By Bantam Books, 1975
- Fasting as a Way of Life, By Allan Cott Published By Bantam Books, 1977
- Healing Crisis through Eliminating Diets and Detoxification, By Bernard Jensen, D.C. (BiWorld Publishers) 1976
- Make Your Juicer Your Drug Store, by Dr. L. Newman, (New York: Benedict Lust Publ), 1970
- How Juices Restore Health Naturally, by Salem Kirnan, (Pennsylvania; Salem Kirban Publisher), 1980
- Fighting Radiation & Chemical Pollutants, By Steven R. Schecter, N.D. (Vitality Ink Pub.) 1988
- The New Enzyme Catalyst Diet: Amazing Way to Quick, Permanent Weight Loss, by Carlson Wade (Parker Publishing)
- The Book of Miso, by William Shurtleff & Akiko Aoyagi (Kanagawa-Ken, Japan; Autumn Press Inc.), 1976
- Massageworks: A Practical Encyclopedia of Massage Techniques, by D. Baloti Lawrence and Lewis Harrison, (New York; The Putnum Publishing Group), 1983
- The Wellness Workbook, by Regina Sara Ryan and John W. Travis M.D., (California; Ten Speed Press), 1981
- Arthritis Can Be Cured, by Bernard Aschner, M.D., (New York; The Julian Press), 1957
- The Book of Whole Grains, by Marlene Anne Bumgarner, (New York, St. Martins Press), 1976
- Dr. Lynch's Holistic Self-Health Program: Three Months to

Total Well-Being, by James P. B. Lynch, D.C. with Anita Weil Bell, (New York; Penguin Books), 1994

• Fighting Radiation and Chemical Pollutants with Foods, Herbs, & Vitamins, (California, Vitality, Ink), 1990

• The New Enzyme-Catalyst Diet: Amazing Way to Quick Permanent Weight Loss, by Carlson Wade, (New York, Parker Publishing Company Inc.), 1976

• The East/West Exercise Book, by David Smith, (New York, McGraw-Hill), 1976

• Food Combining and Digestion, by Steve Meyerowitz, (Massachusetts; The Spout House Inc.), 1993

• Sprout It!, by Steve Meyerowitz, (Massachusetts; The Sprout House Inc.), 1993

• Alternative Healing and Your Health, by J. Maya Pinkington and the Diagram Group, (New York, Ballantine Books), 1991

• The Low-Fat Way to Health and Longer Life, by Lester M. Morrison, M.D., (New Jersey, Prentice Hall), 1958

# INDEX